# CHAIR
# YOGA
## FOR MEN OVER 50

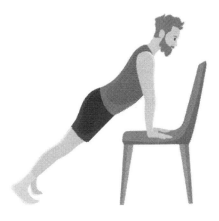

# EMERSON BLAKE

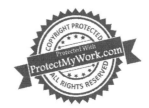

# Contents

# SPECIAL BONUS

As a special bonus for purchasing this book, you can download this **Free Tracking Journal** to accompany your chair yoga journey. This downloadable journal is yours to use as you progress through the book and begin practicing the chair yoga routines.

In the journal you'll find templates to record your experiences, reflections, and progress over time. Use it to set intentions before each session and make notes about how you felt during and after your chair yoga practice. This journal will become a personal keepsake, allowing you to look back on your growth and moments of self-discovery.

Be sure to download and print out this free bonus to enrich your overall chair yoga experience!

# Introduction

You are 50, but that doesn't mean you have to be a passive observer of your life. You are still here, you can still participate, be here now, fully and with intention. These pages that are to follow are not just an introduction to chair yoga; they are an invitation to reclaim your vitality, your life, the very essence of who you were and have always been; to embrace a practice that understands and respects the journey your body has been through.

Too often, society subtly suggests that with age comes an inevitable decline, a slow stepping back from the activities we once loved. But you, the one with the book in your hands, are a testament to the contrary. A kind of rebellion. Men over 50 are not on the periphery of life; they are at the heart of it, rich with experiences, wisdom, and an undiminished desire to live fully. This book is specially created for you, for every man who has looked at the second half of life and seen not a sunset but a new dawn.

Chair yoga is a gentle yet profoundly effective form of exercise that has been adapted to be accessible to anyone, regardless of fitness level, flexibility, or the presence of chronic aches and pains. It's yoga that meets you exactly where you are, using nothing but a chair as a support to offer stability and confidence as you explore movement and breath. This isn't about transforming into someone you're not; it's about becoming the best version of the person you already are.

In these pages to come, you'll learn that chair yoga is more than just a series of stretches and poses. It's a pathway to better health, a means of reducing stress, and a method of finding joy in movement again. It's a form of meditation in action, where each breath and each gentle stretch can bring you into the present moment, into a state of calm awareness where the rush of life slows down and you can catch your breath. This book is steeped in the knowledge that flexibility isn't just physical. It's mental, it's emotional, and yes, it's spiritual too. This book is the companion that will help you to navigate the changes life brings, to bend without breaking, and to find strength in softness. We're going to look into how this practice can help you improve your balance, enhance your flexibility, strengthen your muscles, and quiet your mind.

Okay, if your eyeballs haven't rolled deeply into your sockets yet, you might be thinking, "Yoga? That's not for me. I'm not flexible enough. It's too late to start." But let me assure you, it's not too late, and you are exactly who chair yoga is for. This practice doesn't ask you to be anything other than yourself. It doesn't require you to touch your toes or twist into pretzel shapes. It simply invites you to start. With the turning of each page, you will find stories of men like you who have found chair yoga a companion for this phase of life. They are men who have decided that age will not define them, men who have chosen to meet the challenges of aging with grace, determination, and an open heart.

When we flip through the last page, you won't just know about chair yoga; you will have experienced its transformative power. You will have learned to listen to your body, to honor its wisdom, and to move in ways that feel good and right for you. And most importantly, you will have taken an important step toward maintaining your independence, your health, and your zest for life.

So welcome. Thank you for choosing me as your partner in yoga, this is the beginning of a new way to age; the beginning of a new way of living.

## Chapter One

# Getting Started With Chair Yoga

I wasn't always interested in chair yoga or anything that related to such, but my interest in it developed when a dear friend of mine, Frank, who volunteers at the same foundation as I do, started showing his face on a not-so-regular basis as he usually does. His absence didn't go unnoticed because he was the kind of person who walked into a room and captured the hearts of everyone around. His diminishing presence sparked concern among our circle of friends, and I, the curious person that I am, couldn't help but observe the subtle changes in his demeanor—the lines of pain etched on his face, the weariness in his eyes. It was evident that something was weighing heavily on him, something more than just physical discomfort.

When I had finally mustered the courage to gently ask about his well-being, he opened up and told me about his ongoing battle with chronic back pain. His struggles resonated with me on a personal level, as I, too, had started to experience similar twinges of discomfort because I was also no stranger to the complexities of aging. Frank's story was a poignant reminder of the frailness of our bodies and the importance of prioritizing our health and well-being, especially as we grow older.

Even though he was initially skeptical, he took the leap and decided to explore alternative methods of pain management, which led him to discover the great benefits of chair yoga. Through this gentle yet effective practice, he found relief from his physical discomfort and a renewed sense of vitality that had eluded him for so long. The simple, intentional movements of chair yoga not only alleviated his back pain but also nurtured his emotional and mental well-being, empowering him to reclaim his independence and mobility.

Seeing him heal and reclaim his life inspired me to learn more about the topic. His experience served as a powerful testament to the profound impact that this ancient practice can have on one's overall health and quality of life. Little did I know that by taking that first step, I would not only be opening up a Pandora's box of pleasant surprises, I was planting the very seed that this book sprouted from. I guess life is serendipitous like that, it shows you how one thing can have a positive ripple effect over your life and everything else around you.

## Importance of Heart Health In Men Over 50

Well, I'm going to say it: when you reach the ripe old age of 50, you are no longer a spring chicken. At this stage of life, many men start to become more aware of their health, especially their heart health. The importance of heart health is something that we cannot overstate enough because this demographic is at a higher risk for various heart-related issues. Understanding why these issues become prevalent is crucial for taking proactive steps to maintain a healthy heart.

As you age, there are several factors that contribute to the increased prevalence of heart health issues. One of the primary reasons is the natural aging process itself. As we get older, our blood vessels tend to become less flexible and more prone to plaque buildup, which can lead to conditions such as atherosclerosis. This hardening and narrowing of the arteries restrict blood flow to the heart, increasing the risk of heart attacks and other cardiovascular problems.

In addition to the effects of aging, lifestyle factors play a significant role in heart health. Poor diet, lack of exercise, smoking, excessive alcohol consumption, and high levels of stress can all contribute to the development of heart disease. Men over 50 who have spent years neglecting their health may start to experience the consequences as they age. We are who we are and we come from where we come from so genetics are also bound to factor in as well. A family history of heart disease can significantly increase an individual's risk of developing similar issues. Men with a family history of heart problems should be especially vigilant about monitoring their heart health and taking preventive measures to reduce their risk.

There are hormonal changes that are likely to occur as you age which can impact heart health. Decreased testosterone levels, for example, have been associated with an increased risk of cardiovascular disease. Hormonal imbalances can affect cholesterol levels, blood pressure, and overall heart function, making men more susceptible to heart-related issues as they get older.

Furthermore, underlying health conditions such as high blood pressure, diabetes, obesity, and sleep apnea become more prevalent in men over 50 and can significantly

CHAIR YOGA FOR MEN OVER 50

impact heart health. These conditions, if left untreated, can place added stress on the heart and increase the risk of developing cardiovascular problems.

## *Factors Surrounding Heart Health*

Factors surrounding heart health can have a significant impact on your well-being. These factors can influence heart health, including a sedentary lifestyle due to office jobs, back pain, mobility limitations, and the tendency to prioritize the health and well-being of children and spouses over their own.

A sedentary lifestyle, often associated with office jobs and prolonged sitting, can have detrimental effects on heart health. Lack of physical activity often leads to weight gain, high blood pressure, high cholesterol levels, and increased risk of heart disease. If you spend long hours sitting at a desk or in front of a computer, you may find it challenging to incorporate regular exercise into your daily routine, further increasing your risk of heart-related issues.

Back pain is another common factor that can impact heart health in men over 50. It is something that limits your mobility and makes it difficult to engage in physical activities that support heart health, such as exercise and stretching. Additionally, the discomfort and limitations that it causes, can contribute to a sedentary lifestyle, exacerbating the risk of heart disease.

Mobility limitations, whether they are due to back pain, arthritis, or other health conditions, can also hinder men from engaging in regular exercise and physical activity, which in general impacts how you show up in other areas of your life as well as reduced mobility causes muscle weakness, decreased cardiovascular fitness, and weight gain, all of which can negatively affect heart health.

It is also uncommon to put other people first, most of us from a young age have the belief ingrained within us that we so to say, have to pour into other people's cups first before tending to our own to not seem selfish this way of thinking is often what leads to self-neglect, so what do you do? You put off preventive health screenings, ignore symptoms of heart problems, or fail to prioritize healthy lifestyle habits due to your focus on caregiving responsibilities. While caring for loved ones is important, neglecting your own health can have serious consequences, especially when it comes to your heart health.

# The Importance of Mental Health

Just because you are male, it does not mean that you aren't allowed to have feelings or you are not allowed to be intentional and proactive about taking care of the state of your mental health. Your emotional well-being is just as important as everybody else's. It's unfortunate that in our society, men are often expected to suppress their emotions and "tough it out" when faced with difficulties. This can lead to men feeling isolated and alone as if they have nowhere to turn to for support.

As men age, they may encounter more challenges that can take a toll on their emotional health. Retirement, loss of friends or loved ones, physical limitations, and financial stress are just a few examples. It's important to acknowledge that these challenges can impact mental health and emotional well-being.

Chair yoga for men over 60 can be a great way to not only improve physical health but also promote emotional well-being. By taking time to focus on breathing, mindfulness, and relaxation, men can learn to tune in to their thoughts and emotions. This can help them identify when they may need additional support or care.

You must remember that there is no shame in asking for help. Especially if it is related to your mental health. It is not a sign of weakness, but rather a sign of innate strength. In fact, it takes courage to recognize when you need assistance and to take steps toward improving your mental health. you may feel hesitant to seek support, but there are many resources available to help. From counseling to support groups to online resources, there are many options available to remind you that you are not alone.

## *The Connection Between Mental Well-Being and the Motivation to Prioritize Health*

Mental health is the reserve that you can tap into to find the ultimate enjoyment for life; it is the vehicle that drives our vitality for life; the foundation for our overall well-being and affects how we perceive and prioritize our physical health. When our mental health is in good shape, we are more likely to have the motivation to prioritize our health in general. Here's a breakdown of the connection between mental well-being and the motivation to prioritize health:

It keeps us in touch with our emotions and helps with emotional regulation. Emotional regulation is our ability to notice and be with whatever it is that we are feeling without judgment: This means that you can manage stress, anxiety, and other negative emotions in healthier ways. For example, someone who is in good mental health might use exercise as a tool to cope with stress, thereby prioritizing their physical health to support their mental well-being.

Mental well-being is closely linked to self-efficacy, which is the belief in your ability to achieve goals. When individuals feel good mentally, they are more likely to believe that they can make positive changes in their lives, including adopting healthier habits, they are less likely to be dragged down by the limiting beliefs that try to hold them prisoner and stuck in a constant cycle of self-sabotage. This self-efficacy can drive motivation to prioritize health through actions like consistent exercise, balanced nutrition, or regular health check-ups.

The mind and body are intricately connected, the one cannot exist without the other because they influence each other in various ways. Positive mental health allows you to be aware of and in tune with your body's nuanced needs and signals. For instance, someone in a good mental state may be more attuned to how certain foods make them feel or how exercise impacts their mood. This awareness can drive a person to prioritize activities that support their overall well-being.

Meaning and purpose are what drive our everyday lives. Mental well-being often aligns with a sense of purpose and meaning in life. When you feel fulfilled and purposeful, you are more likely to take care of yourself to continue pursuing your passions and goals. For instance, a person who values quality time with loved ones will prioritize their health to ensure they can show up fully and wholeheartedly for those they love.

Lastly, mental well-being plays a crucial role in sustaining motivation and resilience when facing challenges. Life is hardly easy, there are countless challenges that often threaten to shake the steady foundation of our lives that we're trying to establish. By maintaining good mental health, you become more equipped and resourced to handle setbacks and obstacles on your health journey. This ability to bounce back can fuel the drive to prioritize health, knowing that it contributes to your ability to make it out of those brief periods in the wilderness.

While chair yoga may not be a cure-all solution for all of our mental and physical health issues, it can certainly be a powerful tool in addressing many of these challenges. When you put mindfulness, relaxation techniques, and physical movement, you are saying yes to you, you're saying yes to life. 50, or even 60 years old does not have to mean the end of your life; there's still a whole lot of life to live and you deserve to give yourself the very best of it.

We owe it to ourselves and future generations to continue breaking down the stigma surrounding men's emotional health and encouraging men to prioritize their emotional well-being. Advocating for a culture that values and supports men's mental health is how we can collectively help to reduce the barriers that prevent men from seeking help.

# Chapter Two

# Safety Mindset, and Benefits of Chair Yoga

When I was a teenager we had a gardener named Jim Alesinyole originally from Nigeria. He was as wise as they come and had this rich, metaphorical, and lyrical way of speaking. On one occasion, I recall talking to him about needing to do something but at that time, I wasn't exactly in the right headspace, I remember him looking at me while printing my mothers petunia shrubs, "Emerson," he said looking at me stent, "Even the best cooking pot will not produce food by itself." He continued, "It's the same with everything in life. You can have the best tools, the best resources, and the best conditions, but if your mindset is not in the right place, you won't be able to achieve your goals. You need a safety mindset, a mindset that puts your well-being first, that values progress over perfection, and that understands that ego can often derail progress, especially in men."

Jim's words stayed with me throughout my life. As I transitioned through the various stages of life, I realized that his message was more relevant than ever. Chair yoga is a practice that requires a safety mindset, one that prioritizes the well-being of the practitioner over everything else. It's easy to get caught up in the idea of perfection, to push ourselves too hard, and to let our egos take over, without realizing that in doing so, we risk injury, burnout, and ultimately, not reaching our full potential.

That's why in this chapter, we'll explore the benefits of chair yoga and how to cultivate a safety mindset. We'll look at how to create ideal conditions for chair yoga practice, how to approach the practice with a beginner's mind, and how to let go of the ego that can often hold us back.

# The Benefits of Chair Yoga

Now I know that we've touched on some of the benefits that chair yoga has for you, but we haven't really gone deeply into detail about what those benefits actually are. So let's start off by getting a little into detail about how chair yoga can help us in the various aspects of our lives.

- **Emotional Regulation**: Emotional regulation is your ability to be your emotions. It's having the language and the vocabulary to name your fears, your anxieties, your sadness, frustrations, joy, and everything else in between. It's about learning and teaching ourselves that there's no shame in any emotion; the emotions are merely a part of who we are and we ought to do the best we can to be with them as they surface. Chair yoga helps to regulate emotions by reducing anxiety and depression and promoting feelings of peace and relaxation. This is achieved through controlled breathing, meditation, and physical movements that stimulate the production of endorphins which are feel-good hormones.

- **Stress Relief:** Lie stuff gets in the way and when that happens the tension will usually show up somewhere in our bodies. Chair yoga helps to relieve stress by reducing tension in the body and calming the mind. This helps to lower blood pressure and heart rate, which in turn reduces the risk of heart disease and stroke.

- **Pain Management:** There's nothing worse than living with chronic, unwanted pain. Chair yoga helps to manage that pain by increasing blood flow and oxygenation, which helps to reduce inflammation and promote healing. The gentle movements also help to stretch and strengthen muscles, which can alleviate pain and improve range of motion.

- **Improved Mobility and Flexibility:** Chair yoga helps to improve mobility and flexibility by increasing joint mobility and range of motion. This can help to prevent injuries and improve overall physical function.

- **Confidence**: Chair yoga helps to build confidence by providing a safe and supportive environment where men can challenge themselves physically and mentally. It helps you to tap into power in your body that you had known existed, in a way it reminds you that your body is this breathing, remarkable thing that is capable of doing so, so much.

In addition to these benefits, chair yoga is a great opportunity for you to socialize and connect. This is particularly important because, at 50, you can get incredibly lonely, and knowing that you have people whom you can share that sense of connectedness with can be life-changing for you.

## *Safety Guidelines and Modifications*

Consulting with a healthcare professional before beginning your yoga practice is essential, especially if you are someone who has pre-existing health conditions because your healthcare providers can offer personalized recommendations to ensure that the yoga practice is safe and effective for each of your individual's unique needs.

For instance, let's just say that you are a patient with a history of osteoporosis, if you involve and consult with the healthcare provider, you will receive guidance on modifying poses to protect your bone health and prevent fractures. You will get recommendations on gentle movements that promote strength and flexibility without compromising bone integrity. Also on the same note as well, those with conditions like arthritis, diabetes, or chronic pain can benefit from seeking professional advice before starting chair yoga. Healthcare professionals have enough knowledge that they can share with you on how you can make the practice as safe as possible for you, you'll be able to adapt poses to accommodate joint stiffness, manage blood sugar levels during practice, and incorporate relaxation techniques to alleviate pain and stress.

I guess it might be an extra bit of admin and so forth, but by making sure that you have that solid foundation established before you start the journey, you reduce your risk of exacerbating existing conditions or sustaining injuries. This proactive approach not only safeguards your well-being but also enhances the therapeutic benefits of yoga, fostering a positive and empowering experience.

## *Recommendations for Creating a Safe Environment*

Make sure that the chair is sturdy enough, it's time to bring out the best chair in the house. When practicing chair yoga, you need to make sure you choose a chair that is sturdy and stable, so that you are provided with the necessary support you need for various poses and movements, ensuring that the chair remains secure and safe throughout your practice. The last thing that you need to worry about is having a chair break into a million pieces in the middle of your practice.

You need to practice on a non-slip surface as well. It's important for your safety to practice on a non-slip surface, such as a yoga mat or carpet. This will help prevent the chair from sliding or moving unexpectedly, allowing you to focus on your practice without worrying about stability. To add to this as well, make sure that the soles of your shoes are the correct material and fit.

Create a safe practice area by keeping it clean and free of clutter. Remove any and everything that feels unnecessary to have around, the ids and grandkids' toys, etc. Clearing the space around your chair will reduce the risk of tripping hazards, ensuring a smooth and uninterrupted yoga session for you.

Take the time to adjust the height of your chair to ensure proper alignment during your practice. This will help you maintain good posture, support your spine, and prevent strain on your joints and muscles as you move through different poses. You want to be able to move as freely as possible without feeling like you are enclosed in a box. Make sure there is enough space around your chair for comfortable movement. Having room to extend your arms and legs freely will allow you to transition between poses smoothly and safely, without any obstructions.

A bright well-lit room is your best friend in this instance. To practice chair yoga safely, ensure that your practice area is well-lit. Having mood lighting will help you see your surroundings clearly, reducing the risk of accidents or strain on your eyes during your practice sessions.

## *Listening To Your Body*

Your body will always give you cues and signals that you should listen to. It will always tell you if you are doing too much or, in some cases, too little. When you intentionally take time to tune in and pay attention to these messages, you are respecting your body's limitations and avoiding pain or injury during your chair yoga practice, you are essentially saying and acknowledging, "I know, I can do it, but I'm still respecting the boundaries that my body cannot cross."

Your body is going to have reactions to the different movements and poses throughout the practice. That's what makes it incredibly crucial to be mindful of how your body responds to each movement and pose. If you feel any discomfort, strain, or sharp pain, it's a sign that you may be pushing yourself beyond your current abilities. Ignoring these signals can lead to injuries and setbacks, hindering your progress and enjoyment of the practice.

Listening to your body is all about honoring where you are in the present moment. It's about acknowledging that your body is unique and has its own set of strengths and limitations. Accepting and respecting these boundaries is how you can tailor your practice to suit your individual needs, gradually building strength, flexibility, and balance over time.

Respecting your body's cues, on the other hand, is about making self-compassion a big part of your practice. You are not a robot or a machine that is designed to go for hours on end, you need your rest, your moments of pause where you can catch a break in between all that you are doing. So yes, it's okay to take breaks, modify poses, or skip certain movements if they cause discomfort. Remember that chair yoga is a personal journey, and there is no competition or comparison with others. All that matters is the fact that you are showing up and doing the best that you can. Embrace the idea and the truth that leading yourself with kindness is what will make it easier and more sustainable to navigate your practice.

Also keep in mind that listening to your body fosters a deeper connection between your physical sensations, emotions, and thoughts, which is after all what yoga is about. You owe it to yourself to cultivate that level of so greater body awareness and mindfulness, that you can enhance the mind-body connection; staying attuned to your body's feedback in this way will help you make informed decisions that support your well-being and promote a sustainable and fulfilling experience.

## Physical Considerations

If you want to get the best and the most out of the practice, you're going to need to learn how to do certain things right. I mean just think about it: a long-distance runner needs to have the right form to prevent injuries and run efficiently. Similarly, in chair yoga, paying attention is key to physical considerations that can significantly enhance the benefits of your practice:

- **Posture**: Maintaining good posture is needed for overall well-being. Proper posture helps in aligning the body correctly, reducing strain on muscles and joints, and improving breathing and circulation.

- **Balance**: As we age, balance tends to decline, making us more prone to falls and injuries. Chair yoga can help improve balance by strengthening core muscles and enhancing proprioception, which is your body's sense of its position in space.

- **Alignment**: Correct alignment in yoga poses is crucial to avoid unnecessary stress on joints and muscles. Proper alignment helps in maximizing the benefits of each pose and reduces the risk of injury.

- **Flexibility**: Flexibility is key to maintaining the range of motion in joints and preventing stiffness. Chair yoga can help improve flexibility by gently stretching muscles and increasing mobility in the spine, shoulders, hips, and other key areas.

- **Strength**: Building strength is important for overall health and functional independence. Chair yoga poses can target different muscle groups, helping to improve strength in the arms, legs, core, and back.

- **Awareness of breath**: Focusing on the breath is a fundamental aspect of yoga practice. Deep breathing techniques used in chair yoga can help reduce stress, increase oxygen flow to the brain and body, and promote relaxation.

## *Maintaining Proper Alignment*

Your alignment can be your make or break, the difference between landing up in the hospital because of an injury,  or going back to enjoy the fullness of your life with the same vitality and spark that you had a couple of years back. Here are detailed explanations of how to maintain proper alignment in seated poses:

- **Foundation**: Start by creating a stable and steady foundation. Sit evenly on your chair with both feet flat on the floor, hip-width apart. Distribute your weight evenly between both hips to avoid leaning to one side. Your spine should be in a neutral position, neither slouched nor overly arched.

- **Pelvis**: Align your pelvis in a neutral position by gently engaging your core muscles. Avoid tucking your tailbone under or sticking it out too far. Imagine your pelvis as a bowl of water—keep it level to maintain a stable base of support for your spine.

- **Spine**: Lengthen your spine upward by imagining a string pulling you gently from the crown of your head. This elongation helps in maintaining good posture and prevents unnecessary strain on the back. Avoid rounding or overarching your spine; instead, aim for a natural, relaxed curve.

- **Shoulders**: Relax your shoulders down and back, away from your ears. Avoid hunching or shrugging your shoulders forward, as this can lead to tension in the neck and upper back. Keeping the shoulders relaxed and open allows for better breathing and circulation.

- **Neck**: Align your neck with the rest of your spine by gently tucking your chin and lengthening the back of your neck. Avoid jutting your chin forward or dropping your head back, which can strain the neck muscles and compress the cervical spine.

- **Breath:** Pay attention to your breath as you maintain alignment in seated poses. Deep, steady breathing can help you relax into the poses and improve oxygen flow to your muscles, enhancing the benefits of your practice.

## Tips for Adapting Poses

Just because it's hard does not mean it's impossible. When it comes to things like stiffness, limited flexibility, or reduced mobility, there are various strategies and equipment that you can use to make the process that much more accessible and enjoyable for yourself. Here are some suggestions on what you can do and the equipment you can use to accommodate these challenges.

- **Modify your poses**: You are allowed to modify traditional yoga poses to suit your individual needs and abilities. For example, if a full forward bend is challenging due to stiffness, you can perform a seated forward fold with the support of a chair. Making these slight modifications allows you to experience the benefits of yoga while working within your limitations.

- **Incorporate props**: Props such as yoga blocks, straps, and bolsters can be incredibly helpful in chair yoga practice. Blocks can be used to bring the floor closer to the hands in seated poses, while straps can assist in stretching tight muscles. Bolsters will also provide support and comfort during relaxation poses, promoting a sense of ease and relaxation.

- **Chair variation**: Experimenting with different chair variations can cater to various levels of flexibility and mobility. You can alternate between a sturdy chair with or without armrests, a folding chair, or a chair with a cushion for added comfort. Choosing the right chair can provide stability and support during poses.

- **Focus on breath**: Connection to your breath is a key aspect of yoga (an exercise in general) If you battle with stiffness or limited mobility, deep, mindful breathing throughout the practice will enhance relaxation, reduce stress, and increase oxygen flow to muscles and joints.

- **Move gently**: One of the biggest misconceptions that we have is that for exercise to be effective, it has to be hardcore but incorporating gentle movements and flowing sequences helps improve flexibility and mobility gradually. Go ahead and explore gentle twists, side stretches, and slow, controlled movements to increase the range of motion and release tightness in muscles.

- **Be consistent and patient**: Progress requires time and consistency, you are not going to see any results instantly, but after a week or so yes, you definitely will. Be patient with yourself and listen to your body, if your body tells you that it's had enough at the 15-minute mark, go ahead and stop; 15 minutes is better than nothing. Showing up consistently, even in small increments, can lead to significant improvements in flexibility, mobility, and overall well-being over time. Rome wasn't built in a day, so it's hardly fair to you to expect you to go full force and expect to see results in a couple of hours. My runners say that forward is a pace, keep that in mind as well.

## *Mindfulness and Self-Care*

Self-care and mindfulness are all about noticing. Noticing how you feel, how you're doing, it's those moments and spaces in between time where you can just settle in and be still. Still enough to feel the rise and fall of your breath, steady and rhythmic, a constant anchor amidst life's ever-changing tides. When you're deep in your chair yoga practice, learn to pay attention to each movement, each stretch, each sensation that arises within your body. This practice encourages you to be present in the moment, letting go of past worries and future concerns.

Incorporating self-care into your daily routine is a way of nurturing your well-being, and your physical and mental health. When you take this time to focus on yourself, you are honoring your body and mind, recognizing the importance of balance and harmony in your life. Mindfulness allows you to cultivate a sense of awareness, bringing attention to your thoughts and feelings without judgment or attachment. This non-reactive awareness can help you navigate challenges with clarity and composure. Self-care is not a luxury but a necessity, as necessary as the very air that you are breathing. It is something that allows you to recharge, rejuvenate, and realign yourself, promoting a sense of inner peace and tranquility. Choosing to prioritize your well-being makes you feel more resourced to face the demands of daily life with resilience and grace. Self-care and mindfulness go hand in hand, guiding you toward a deeper understanding of yourself and your place in the world.

So, welcome and embrace these moments of stillness, these opportunities to connect with your inner self, and weave them into the very fabric of your being. Believe me when I say that they will change you and your life.

## *Incorporating Relaxation Techniques*

Relaxation techniques play a key role in chair yoga, they offer a sanctuary for the mind and body to unwind and rejuvenate. One such technique is deep breathing, where you focus on slow, deep breaths that fill your lungs completely. This practice calms the nervous system, lowers stress levels, and promotes a sense of relaxation. Incorporating deep breathing into chair yoga sessions can help center your mind and energize your body simultaneously.

Another effective relaxation technique is progressive muscle relaxation. This method involves tensing each muscle group in your body for a few seconds and then releasing the tension, allowing the muscles to relax fully. As you practice progressive muscle relaxation during chair yoga, you become more attuned to the subtle sensations in your body, fostering a deeper mind-body connection, this technique not only relieves physical tension but also promotes mental clarity and focus.

Visualization is yet another technique that can be integrated into the practice. When you close your eyes and imagine a peaceful, serene place, such as a tranquil beach or a lush forest, you create a mental escape from everyday stressors. Visualization helps reduce anxiety, enhances concentration, and cultivates a positive outlook.

Mindful meditation is another effective relaxation technique that strengthens the mind and body simultaneously. The focus on the present moment, free of judgment, builds mindfulness, awareness, and acceptance. Mindful meditation during chair yoga helps quiet the mind, reduce distractions, and enhance mental resilience. This practice fosters a sense of balance and inner harmony, promoting overall mental and physical wellness.

# Chapter Three

# Warm-Up And Breathing Techniques

So I'm going to be upfront and honest: I wasn't always the kind of person to do my warm-ups before exercising or doing movement of any kind. When I went through my "I'm going to be a long-distance runner" phase, which everyone seems to go through at some point in their lives. I remember just going for it before races, no stretches, in between, nothing. I guess I thought I was Invincible.

All of that changed through one fall at the local park. I was there at the starting line with a pool of other eager faces, all of us ready to tackle the half-marathon ahead. The energy was rich and palpable, and the excitement was buzzing through like electricity. There, I bounced off the balls of my feet, cool air filling my lungs, and oh, I felt unstoppable.

The starting gun went off and we all headed off, all of us in a stampede of determination and spandex. The first couple of mines were a breeze. My strides were even and my breathing steady, the rhythm of my footsteps echoing like a well-oiled machine. When I reached mile seven, though, something felt slightly off.

It started off as a nagging twinge in my left knee, a small discomfort that I brushed aside. I told myself that it was nothing, just a passing kind of pain that would vanish as quickly as it came, but as I progressed through each mile, I could no longer bear that pain. When I reached mile nine, I was hobbling, the pain searing through my knee with every step I took. The realization hit me with the force of a sledgehammer: I was injured. And worse, I was injured because I had neglected the most basic principle of physical activity - the warm-up.

As I limped to the sideline, my race over, the weight of what had happened really began to sink in. I watched as other runners, many of them older and wiser, continued the race I could no longer finish. Many of them had spent a good half hour or more before the race stretching and warming up their muscles. They understood something I had failed to grasp—that our bodies are not indestructible, and that preparation is key. The weeks that followed were a flurry of doctor's appointments, physical therapy sessions, and a growing sense of frustration. Gone were the days of spontaneous runs and the pride of finishing races. In their place were ice packs, knee braces, and a slow, humbling journey back to mobility.

I found a silver lining, though, As part of my rehabilitation, my therapist introduced me to chair yoga. At first, I was skeptical. Yoga was for the flexible, the calm, the ones who had their life together—not for a stubborn runner nursing an injured knee. But as I practiced, I noticed something miraculous. Not only did my knee begin to heal, but my entire body started to feel stronger, more resilient, and. most shockingly, more flexible.

As I reshare this experience with you, I do so with the utmost amount of respect for the importance of warm-ups and breathing techniques. They aren't just preludes. They are the foundation upon which all good movement is built. While I may have learned the lesson the hard way, you certainly don't have to. I hope that I can pass on this important lesson to you, a lesson that I now carry into every aspect of my life.

## Simple Breathing Exercises

If you want to be fully engaged in your practice you need to learn to be one with your breath and allow your breath to be one with you. You might be panicking; thinking that this is going to be absolutely impossible to do, but it isn't. You can teach yourself. I've got a couple of breathing exercises that are easy to follow here they are:

### Deep Belly Breathing Exercise with a Chair

This is an exercise that can help you release any excess stress that you're holding onto. It'll help you relax, clear your mind, and settle into the practice

1. Position yourself comfortably on a chair with your feet flat on the ground and your hands resting on your thighs.

2. Close your eyes and take a few deep breaths, inhaling through your nose and exhaling through your mouth. Allow yourself to relax and let go of any tension in your body.

3. Place one hand on your belly and the other on your chest. Take a deep breath

in through your nose, feeling your belly expand as you inhale.

4. Hold your breath for a few seconds, and then exhale slowly through your mouth, feeling your belly contract as you exhale.

5. Repeat this deep belly breathing exercise for several minutes, focusing on your breath and allowing yourself to fully relax.

6. As you continue to breathe deeply, try to extend your exhale so that it is longer than your inhale. This can help to further calm your mind and reduce stress.

7. If you find that your mind starts to wander, gently bring your attention back to your breath and the sensation of your belly rising and falling with each inhale and exhale.

8. When you are ready to end the exercise, take a few more deep breaths, feeling the energy and relaxation that you have generated in your body and mind.

## Counted Breath Exercise with a Chair

1. Sit comfortably on a chair with your feet flat on the ground and your hands resting on your thighs.

2. Close your eyes and take a few deep breaths, inhaling through your nose and exhaling through your mouth. Allow yourself to relax and let go of any tension in your body.

3. When you feel ready, begin to count your breaths. Inhale deeply through your nose and count "one", hold your breath for a few seconds, and then exhale slowly through your mouth, counting "two".

4. Inhale again deeply through your nose, counting "three", hold your breath for a few seconds, and then exhale slowly through your mouth, counting "four".

5. Continue this pattern of counting your breaths, inhaling for a count of "five", holding for a few seconds, and then exhaling for a count of "six".

6. As you continue to count your breaths, try to make each inhale and exhale long and smooth. Focus your attention on your breath and the counting, allowing yourself to fully relax.

7. If you find that your mind starts to wander, gently bring your attention back to your breath and the counting.

8. Continue this counted breath exercise for several minutes, or for as long as feels comfortable for you.

9. When you are ready to end the exercise, take a few more deep breaths, feeling the energy and relaxation that you have generated in your body and mind.

## Alternate Nostril Breathing

Also known as Nadi Shodhana, is a type of breathing exercise that can help calm the mind, reduce stress, and improve overall well-being. Here are step-by-step instructions for performing this breathing exercise with a chair as a prop:

1. Sit on a chair with your spine straight and your feet flat on the ground.

2. Place your left hand on your left knee, palm facing up.

3. Bring your right hand up to your face, and position your index and middle fingers between your eyebrows.

4. Use your right thumb to close your right nostril, and inhale deeply through your left nostril.

5. Once you've inhaled fully, use your ring finger to close your left nostril, and exhale completely through your right nostril.

6. Inhale deeply through your right nostril, then use your right thumb to close your right nostril and exhale completely through your left nostril.

7. Continue this process, alternating between nostrils after each inhale, for several rounds or as long as you feel comfortable.

8. When you're ready to finish, take one final exhale through your left nostril, then lower your hand back down to your left knee and take a few normal breaths before opening your eyes.

Remember to breathe deeply and slowly throughout the exercise, and to keep your movements gentle and fluid. With practice, you may find that alternate nostril breathing becomes a useful tool for managing stress and promoting relaxation

## Sama Vritti

Also known as Equal Breathing, is a simple yet powerful breathing technique that can help to calm the mind, reduce stress, and promote relaxation. Here are step-by-step instructions for performing this technique with a chair as a prop:

1. Sit comfortably in a chair with your spine straight and your feet flat on the ground.

2. Place your hands on your knees, palms facing up or down, whichever feels more comfortable for you.

3. Close your eyes and take a few deep breaths, inhaling through your nose and exhaling through your mouth. Allow yourself to relax and let go of any tension in your body.

4. Begin to inhale and exhale through your nose, making each inhale and exhale the same length.

5. If it helps, you can count the length of your breaths. For example, you might inhale for a count of four, and then exhale for a count of four.

6. As you continue to breathe in this way, try to make each inhale and exhale long and smooth. Focus your attention on your breath, allowing yourself to fully relax.

7. If you find that your mind starts to wander, gently bring your attention back to your breath and the counting.

8. Continue this equal breathing exercise for several minutes, or for as long as feels comfortable for you.

9. When you are ready to end the exercise, take a few more deep breaths, feeling the energy and relaxation that you have generated in your body and mind.

Doing this regularly will help to reduce stress, improve your focus and concentration, and promote a sense of calm and relaxation. The chair can be used as a prop to help you sit with a straight spine and maintain good posture, which can enhance the effectiveness of the exercise.

## Part Breath

Part Breath is a breathing exercise that can help to calm the mind, reduce stress, and promote relaxation. Here are step-by-step instructions for performing this technique with a chair as a prop:

1. Sit comfortably on a chair with your back straight and your feet flat on the ground. Rest your hands on your thighs.

2. Take a few deep breaths, inhaling through your nose and exhaling through your mouth. Allow yourself to relax and let go of any tension in your body.

3. Place your right hand on your belly and your left hand on your chest.

4. Inhale deeply through your nose, feeling your belly expand as you inhale. Allow the breath to fill your belly, ribcage, and chest.

5. Hold your breath for a few seconds, and then exhale slowly through your mouth, feeling your chest, ribcage, and belly contract as you exhale.

6. Repeat this deep, full breath for several rounds, focusing on the sensation of the breath moving through your body.

7. As you continue to breathe deeply, try to make each inhale and exhale long and smooth. Focus your attention on your breath and the sensation of your hands rising and falling with each inhale and exhale.

8. If you find that your mind starts to wander, gently bring your attention back to your breath and the sensation of your hands on your body.

9. Continue this breath exercise for several minutes, or for as long as feels comfortable for you.

10. When you are ready to end the exercise, take a few more deep breaths, feeling the energy and relaxation that you have generated in your body and mind.

## Warm-Up Exercises

Warm-up exercises are an essential part of any workout routine, including chair yoga. The purpose of warming up is to prepare your body for the physical activity ahead by gradually increasing your heart rate, breathing rate, and blood flow to your muscles.

By doing so, you improve the flexibility and mobility of your joints, reduce the risk of injury, and enhance your performance during the workout.

Skipping warm-up exercises can result in muscle strains, sprains, and other injuries, which can ultimately hinder your fitness progress. Although it may add a few extra minutes to your workout, the benefits of warming up greatly outweigh the time it takes. So, it's important to always make time for a proper warm-up before engaging in any physical activity, no matter how intense or mild it may be.

## Seated Cat-Cow

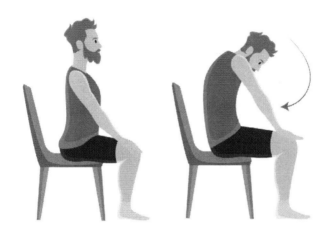

Seated Cat-Cow is an excellent warm-up exercise to help loosen up your spine and improve your posture.

1. Sit upright in your chair with your feet flat on the ground, hip-width apart, and your hands resting on your thighs.

2. Inhale slowly and deeply, bringing your shoulders up towards your ears while simultaneously arching your back and lifting your chest.

3. Hold this position for a few seconds, feeling the stretch in your spine and chest.

4. Exhale slowly and deeply, bringing your shoulders down and rounding your spine forward while tucking your chin to your chest.

5. Hold this position for a few seconds, feeling the stretch in your upper back and neck.

6. Repeat this movement, inhaling as you arch your back and exhaling as you round your spine forward. Move slowly and mindfully, focusing on the

sensations in your body.

7. Continue for 10-15 repetitions, or until you feel adequately warmed up.

Remember to breathe deeply and slowly throughout the exercise, and move at a pace that feels comfortable for you. Seated Cat-Cow is a gentle warm-up exercise that can be modified to suit your needs, so feel free to adjust the movements as necessary.

## Seated Side-Stretch

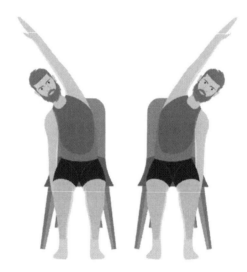

Seated Side-Stretch is a great warm-up exercise to loosen up your side muscles and improve your breathing.

1. Sit upright in your chair with your feet flat on the ground, hip-width apart, and your hands resting on your thighs.

2. Inhale slowly and raise your left arm, reaching your fingertips towards the ceiling.

3. Exhale slowly and lean your torso to the right, keeping your left arm extended overhead.

4. Hold this position for a few seconds, feeling the stretch along the left side of your body.

5. Inhale and return to the starting position with your left arm at your side.

6. Repeat the movement on the opposite side, raising your right arm and leaning your torso to the left.

7. Hold this position for a few seconds, feeling the stretch along the right side of your body.

8. Inhale and return to the starting position.

9. Continue alternating sides for 10-15 repetitions, or until you feel adequately warmed up.

Remember to keep your shoulders relaxed and your spine straight throughout the exercise. Breathe deeply and slowly throughout the movement, focusing on the stretch in your side muscles. Seated Side-Stretch is a gentle warm-up exercise that can be modified to suit your needs, so feel free to adjust the movements as necessary.

## Seated Twist

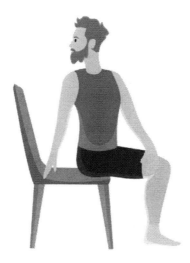

Seated Twist is an excellent warm-up exercise to help loosen up your spine and improve your digestion.

1. Sit upright in your chair with your feet flat on the ground, hip-width apart, and your hands resting on your thighs.

2. Inhale slowly and sit up tall, lengthening your spine.

3. Exhale slowly and twist your torso to the right, placing your left hand on the outside of your right thigh and your right hand behind you on the chair.

4. Hold this position for a few seconds, feeling the stretch along your spine.

5. Inhale and return to the starting position.

6. Repeat the movement on the opposite side, twisting your torso to the left and placing your right hand on the outside of your left thigh and your left hand behind you on the chair.

7. Hold this position for a few seconds, feeling the stretch along your spine.

8. Inhale and return to the starting position.

9. Continue alternating sides for 10-15 repetitions, or until you feel adequately warmed up.

Remember to move slowly and mindfully throughout the exercise, focusing on the sensations in your body. Keep your shoulders relaxed and your spine straight throughout the movement. Seated Twist is a gentle warm-up exercise that can be modified to suit your needs, so feel free to adjust the movements as necessary.

## Seated Shoulder Rolls

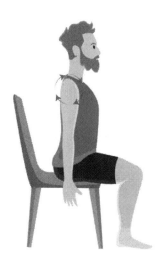

Seated Shoulder Rolls are an excellent warm-up exercise to help loosen up your shoulder muscles and improve your posture.

1. Sit upright in your chair with your feet flat on the ground, hip-width apart, and your hands resting on your thighs.

2. Inhale slowly and lift both shoulders up towards your ears.

3. Exhale slowly and roll your shoulders back and down in a circular motion.

4. Inhale and lift your shoulders up towards your ears again.

5. Exhale and roll your shoulders forward and down in a circular motion.

6. Continue alternating between rolling your shoulders back and down and forward and down in a slow and controlled circular motion.

7. Repeat the movement for 10-15 repetitions, or until you feel adequately warmed up.

Remember to keep your spine straight and your breathing slow and controlled throughout the exercise. Seated Shoulder Rolls is a gentle warm-up exercise that can be modified to suit your needs, so feel free to adjust the movements as necessary.

## Wrist Rolls

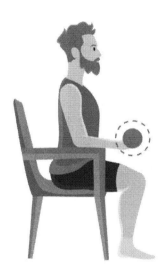

Wrist and Ankle Rolls are great warm-up exercises to help loosen up your wrists and ankles and improve your joint mobility.

1. Sit upright in your chair with your feet flat on the ground, hip-width apart, and your hands resting on your thighs.

2. Extend your arms out in front of you, keeping your elbows straight and your palms facing down.

3. Slowly and gently roll your wrists in a circular motion, rotating your hands clockwise and then counterclockwise.

4. Repeat the movement for 10-15 repetitions, or until you feel adequately warmed up.

## Ankle Rolls

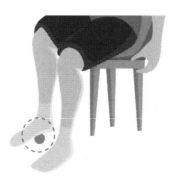

1. Sit upright in your chair with your feet flat on the ground, hip-width apart.

2. Lift your right foot off the ground and slowly and gently roll your ankle in a circular motion, rotating your foot clockwise and then counterclockwise.

3. Repeat the movement with your left foot.

4. Continue alternating between rolling your right ankle and your left ankle for 10-15 repetitions, or until you feel adequately warmed up.

Remember to move slowly and mindfully throughout the exercise, focusing on the sensations in your joints. Wrist and Ankle Rolls are gentle warm-up exercises that can be modified to suit your needs, so feel free to adjust the movements as necessary.

# Chapter Four

# Fundamental Chair Yoga Poses

When I went to India a couple of years back, I met with a yogi who had a presence that seemed to transcend time itself. His eyes held the wisdom of centuries, and his voice carried a serenity that calmed the most restless of minds. I found myself drawn to him like a moth to a flame, eager to soak in even a fraction of the knowledge he possessed. We sat together in the quiet courtyard of his humble ashram, the sounds of nature providing a soothing backdrop to our conversation. As we sipped on steaming cups of chai, he began to share stories of his own journey along the path of yoga, stories that wove together threads of struggle, triumph, and ultimately, enlightenment.

One tale, in particular, struck a chord deep within me. He spoke of a time when he was just a young man, alive with ambition and a thirst for knowledge. He had sought out the guidance of a renowned guru, hoping to unlock the secrets of the universe and his place within it. But instead of imparting grandiose wisdom or esoteric teachings, the guru handed him a simple wooden chair.

Confused and somewhat disappointed, he questioned the guru's choice. What could a chair possibly teach him about the mysteries of life and existence? But the guru had simply smiled and replied, "In this chair, you will find all the answers you seek."

Intrigued by the guru's cryptic words, he had taken the chair to a quiet corner of the ashram and sat down. At first, he fidgeted restlessly, unable to see how a mere piece of furniture could hold any profound truths. But as the hours passed and the sun dipped below the horizon, something within him shifted.

In the stillness of that moment, the young yogi began to observe the chair with new eyes. He noticed its sturdy legs, roots firmly planted in the earth, a reminder of the importance of grounding oneself in the present moment. He traced the curve of its back, a gentle reminder to maintain a straight spine and an open heart in the face of life's challenges. And he felt the smooth surface of its seat, a symbol of the peace that comes from finding stillness within.

As he sat there, lost in contemplation, the young yogi realized that the chair was not just a piece of furniture; it was a mirror reflecting back to him the truths he had been seeking all along. In its simplicity and quiet strength, he found the essence of yoga itself—a practice that is not about contorting the body into impossible shapes or achieving external perfection, but about finding harmony and balance within.

The lessons the yogi had learned from that humble chair had guided him on his own path to enlightenment, and now, as he shared them with me, I felt a spark of recognition ignite within my own heart. At that moment, I understood that true wisdom is not found in the grand gestures or lofty words of sages, but in the quietude of a simple chair and the profound teachings it holds for those willing to listen.

As I left the ashram that day, the words spoken that day echoed in my mind, a gentle reminder that the most fundamental truths are often found in the most unexpected of places. I carried with me the wisdom of that simple wooden chair, a silent teacher whose lessons would shape the rest of the trajectory of my life.

## Fundamental Poses for a Strong Chair Yoga Foundation

As we are about to start, I know we have already discussed tips and stuff but I want to leave you with a few more considerations that you should keep in mind.

1. **Keep your feet grounded:** It's important to keep your feet firmly planted on the ground throughout your practice to maintain stability and prevent injury.

2. **Engage your core:** Engaging your core muscles can help you maintain proper alignment and support your lower back during your practice.

3. **Don't overstretch:** While it's important to stretch and lengthen your muscles, it's equally important not to overstretch or push your body too far. Remember to move slowly and mindfully, and never force yourself into a pose that doesn't feel right

4. **Breathe deeply:** Deep, slow breathing can help you relax and stay focused during your practice. Remember to breathe deeply and evenly throughout your poses.

5. **Stay hydrated:** It's important to stay hydrated before, during, and after your practice to prevent dehydration and keep your body functioning properly.

## Seated Mountain Pose: Tadasana

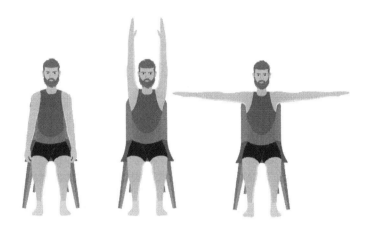

Seated Mountain Pose (Tadasana) is a seated variation of the traditional Mountain Pose. It is a foundational yoga pose that helps to promote good posture, strengthen the core muscles, and calm the mind.

Here are the step-by-step instructions on how to do Seated Mountain Pose:

1. Sit on the edge of a firm chair with your feet planted on the ground and your hands resting loosely at your side.

2. Close your eyes and take a few deep breaths, inhaling through your nose and exhaling through your mouth.

3. Lengthen your spine by elongating your neck and pulling your shoulders back and down.

4. Engage your core muscles by drawing your navel in towards your spine.

5. Keep your feet grounded and gently press your sitting bones down into the chair.

6. Hold the pose for 5-10 deep breaths, and then release.

## Seated Forward Fold: Uttanasana

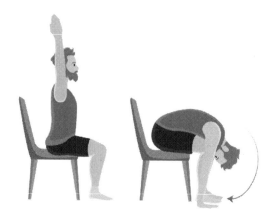

Seated Forward Fold (Uttanasana) pose that helps to stretch and lengthen the muscles of the back, hamstrings, and calves. It also helps to calm the mind and relieve stress. Repeat this 2-3 times at the beginning or end of your practice to help warm up or cool down the body and prepare for more challenging poses.

This is how you do it.

1. Start by sitting on the edge of a chair with your feet planted firmly on the ground.

2. Inhale and lift your arms up towards the ceiling, lengthening your spine.

3. Exhale and fold forward from the hips, keeping your spine long and your neck relaxed.

4. Reach for your feet or ankles, or place your hands on the floor in front of you.

5. Gently pull yourself forward with each exhale, stretching your hamstrings and lengthening your spine.

6. Hold the pose for 5-10 deep breaths, and then release.

## Seated Tree Pose Vrksasana

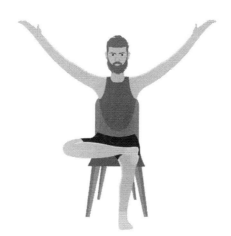

Seated Tree Pose (Vrksasana) is a seated yoga pose that helps to improve balance, concentration, and stability.

1. Start by sitting on a firm chair with your feet planted firmly on the ground.

2. Bend your right knee and place the sole of your foot on the inside of your left thigh, pressing your foot into your thigh.

3. Place your right hand on your right knee and your left hand on your left thigh.

4. Lengthen your spine and engage your core muscles.

5. Inhale and lift your arms up towards the ceiling, keeping your shoulders relaxed.

6. Exhale and bring your hands together in front of your heart, maintaining your balance.

7. Hold the pose for 5-10 deep breaths, and then release.

8. Repeat the pose on the other side, switching the placement of your feet.

Seated Tree Pose can be repeated 2-3 times on each side at the beginning or end of your yoga practice to help improve balance, concentration, and stability.

## Seated Leg Lifts

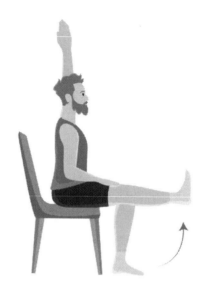

Seated Leg Lifts help to strengthen the core and leg muscles, improve flexibility, and promote good posture.

This is how you are going to do the exercise:

1. Start by sitting on a chair with your feet planted firmly on the ground.

2. Place your hands on the floor beside your hips, fingers pointing towards your feet.

3. Engage your core muscles and keep your back straight.

4. Inhale and lift your right leg up towards the ceiling, keeping your toes pointing towards the sky.

5. Exhale and lower your leg back down to the floor.

6. Repeat the movement with your left leg.

7. Continue alternating legs for 10-15 repetitions.

## Seat Pigeon Pose

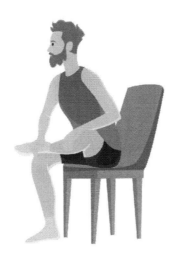

The seated pigeon pose is a hip opener that can be done while seated in a chair. It stretches the outer hips, glutes, and thighs. Here are easy instructions on how you're going to perform this pose:

1. Sit towards the front edge of your chair with your feet flat on the floor, about hip-width apart.

2. Cross your right ankle over your left thigh, bringing your right knee out towards the side as far as is comfortable. Your right calf should be parallel to the front edge of the chair.

3. Keep your left leg stationary, with your left foot flat on the floor.

4. Sit up tall, lengthening through your spine. You can hold onto the sides of the chair for support.

5. Take a few deep breaths, relaxing your hips towards the chair with each exhale.

6. For a deeper stretch, walk your hands forward and fold at the hips, hinging from your hip joints rather than rounding your spine.

7. Hold for 5-8 breaths, then slowly unwind and switch legs.

**Here are some safety tips to remember:**

- Don't force the pose. Only go as far as feels like a comfortable stretch, without pain.

- Use a cushion or folded blanket under your hips if needed to alleviate pressure.

- If you have any knee/hip injuries or conditions, omit or modify this pose based on your doctor's advice.

- Focus on your breathing to relax into the stretch gradually.

## Plank

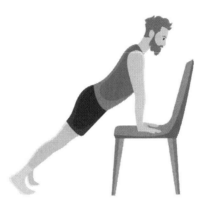

The chair plank is a core-strengthening exercise that is designed to work the abdominals, back, and arms while using a chair for support. It's a modified version of the full plank. This is how you do it:

1. Place a sturdy, armless chair against a wall for stability. Stand facing the back of the chair.

2. Extend your arms and place your hands shoulder-width apart on the seat of the chair. Walk your feet back until your body forms a straight line from heels to head. Engage your core muscles.

3. Make sure your hands are directly under your shoulders and your body is in one long diagonal line from heels to head. Don't let your hips sag or pike up.

4. Hold this plank position, breathing normally, for 30 seconds to start. Work up to holding for 1 minute.

5. To release, walk your feet back in towards the chair.

And always important to remember, some **safety tips**:

- Keep your abs braced and don't let your lower back sag or arch excessively.

- Don't hold your breath. Breathe normally throughout.

- If you have wrist issues, you can make fists with your hands instead of flat palms.

- Don't lock your elbows—keep them soft with a slight bend.

And that's it for this chapter. In the next chapter, we get to the really good stuff. We look into the poses that target back pain and stiffness.

# Chapter Five

# Special Focus Routines–Targeting Back Pain and Stiffness

I love my desk job and I am incredibly grateful for it, but there's something more sinister that comes with the territory of having a sedentary desk job–back pain. It started as a dull ache, barely noticeable at first, just a whisper of discomfort in the background of my daily life. I ignored it, attributing it to stress or maybe a poor night's sleep. But as days turned into weeks, the ache grew into a persistent throb that seemed to have taken up permanent residence in my lower back.

I tried to brush it off, thinking it would go away on its own if I just toughed it out. I mean, I'm a man in my fifties—a little back pain is par for the course, right? But as the pain intensified, spreading its tendrils up my spine and down my legs, I knew I couldn't ignore it any longer.

One morning, as I struggled to tie my shoes, the pain shot through me like a lightning bolt, bringing me to my knees. It was a wake-up call, a stark reminder that I couldn't keep pushing through the pain and pretending everything was fine. Something had to change.

I sought out doctors, chiropractors, physical therapists—anyone who could offer me relief. They all had different theories about what was causing my back pain – poor posture, muscle imbalances, and even the way I slept. But one thing they all agreed on was the importance of movement and flexibility in maintaining a healthy back.

Through trial and error, I discovered the power of yoga—specifically chair yoga tailored for men over 50. As I learned to move mindfully, to stretch and strengthen my body in ways I never had before, I felt the tightness in my back begin to loosen.

The pain didn't disappear overnight, but with each practice, I felt a little more relief and a little more freedom in my body.

I realized that my back pain wasn't just a physical issue—it was a symptom of a life out of balance. Years of sitting at a desk, hunching over a computer, and neglecting my body's need for movement and care had taken its toll. But through yoga, I found a path back to health and vitality, a way to reclaim my body and my life.

So, if you're like me, grappling with back pain and stiffness that seems to have no end in sight, know that there is hope.

## Seated Boat Pose (Navasana)

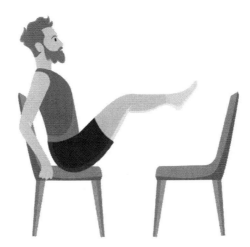

Navasana gets its name from the Sanskrit words "Nava" meaning boat and "Asana" meaning pose. It strengthens your abdominal muscles, hip flexors, and spinal muscles as well as improves balance, posture, and concentration. It's challenging and requires a lot of core engagement and balance, but you can modify it by bending the knees or holding onto the thighs if needed.

1. Sit comfortably on a firm chair with your feet on the ground. You can have a chair in front of you for extra support.

2. Place your hands slightly behind your hips, fingers pointing towards the feet.

3. Engage your core muscles by pulling your navel towards your spine.

4. Lean back slightly and lift your feet off the floor, bringing your shins parallel to the floor.

5. Straighten your legs so they form a 45-degree angle with the floor.

6. Keep your chest lifted, and your back straight.

7. Balance on your sit bones and lengthen through your spine.

8. Extend your arms forward alongside your legs, palms facing each other.

9. Hold the pose for 5-10 breaths, gradually extending the duration as you build strength.

10. To release, lower your feet back to the floor and relax.

## Seated Knee-to-Chest Pose (Apanasana)

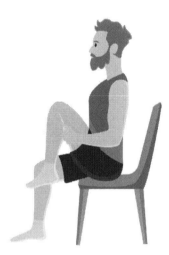

The Seated Knee-to-Chest Pose (Apanasana) is a gentle forward bend that helps stretch the back and release tension. Here's how to do it:

1. Sit on a chair with your legs extended in front of you.

2. Bend your right knee and bring it towards your chest.

3. Clasp your hands around your shins or thighs, and gently pull your knee towards your body.

4. Keep your back straight and your head up, or you can fold forward over your legs if comfortable.

5. Hold the pose for several breaths, then release and repeat on the other side.

**Safety tips for Apanasana:**

1. Go slowly and don't force the stretch. Only bring your knees as close to your chest as is comfortable. Don't bounce or pull too hard.

2. Keep your spine neutral and avoid rounding your back excessively. This could strain the lower back muscles.

3. If you have knee injuries or tightness in the hamstrings, modify by keeping your knees slightly bent or placing a strap/towel around your thighs to hold the pose.

This pose should be gentle and relaxing. Listen to your body and back off if you feel any sharp pain or discomfort. Proper alignment and controlled breathing are key.

## Seated Chair Pose (Utkatasana)

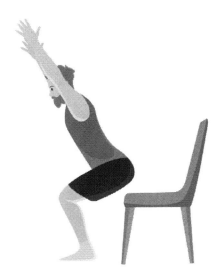

This exercise is a great way to improve posture and relieve back pain and stiffness. It's accessible, and you can modify it to suit your individual needs. The following steps are going to detail how you're going to perform your seated chair pose exercise.

1. Stand close enough to a sturdy chair so that you can sit back on it.

2. You will need to position your feet flat on the ground and make sure that your back is straight. Your feet should be hip-width apart and your toes pointing forward.

3. Place your hands on your knees with your palms facing down.

4. As you inhale a generous amount of air, lift your arms up and extend them towards the ceiling. Keep your shoulders relaxed and your elbows straight.

5. As you exhale and slowly let your breath out, bend your knees and lower your hips towards the chair as if you are sitting down. Make sure your knees are directly over your ankles and your thighs are parallel to the ground.

6. Hold the pose for a few deep breaths, keeping your gaze forward and your core engaged.

7. To come out of the pose, straighten your legs and lower your arms back down to your knees.

Safety is important, so I have added some safety considerations to keep in mind while performing the Seated Chair Pose:

- Make sure you avoid rounding your back or slouching forward. Keep your spine straight and your shoulders relaxed throughout the pose.

- If you experience any discomfort or pain, come out of the pose immediately.

## Seated High Plank Pose (Utthita Chaturanga Dandasana)

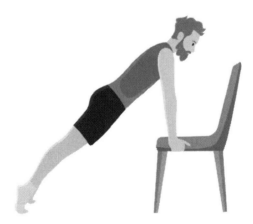

A seated high plank involves holding a high plank position while seated on a chair. Its "Utthita Chaturanga Dandasana" is derived from Sanskrit, where "Utthita" means extended, "Chatur" means four, "Anga" means limb, "Danda" means staff, and "Asana" means pose, essentially the name translates to "Extended Four-Limbed Staff Pose." In doing this pose, you'll be strengthening your core and shoulders while improving your posture as well. This is a challenging one so make modifications as needed.

1. Begin by standing in front of your chair—ensure your chair is backed up against a wall to prevent it from sliding out from under you.

2. Place your hands on the sides of the chair, shoulder-width apart, and step your feet back until your body is in a straight line from head to heels.

3. Slowly raise your body, edging your toes closer to the chair so that you begin to reach an elevated position.

4. Engage your core and hold the pose for a few deep breaths.

5. To release the pose, gently lower your knees to the ground and come back to a seated position.

Some things to keep in mind to ensure that the flow goes as seamlessly as possible

- Keep your shoulders directly over your wrists and your core engaged to maintain proper alignment.

- Avoid letting your hips sag or lifting them too high. Your body should be in a straight line from head to heels.

- Make adjustments as needed if it gets uncomfortable

## Seated Cobra Pose (Bhujangasana)

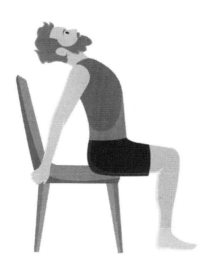

Seated Cobra Pose, also known as Bhujangasana, involves stretching your upper body while seated on a chair. It is derived from Sanskrit, where "Bhujanga" means serpent or snake, and "Asana" means pose.

1. Start in a seated position on a chair with your feet flat on the floor and your hands resting on your thighs.

2. Place your hands on the back of the chair, shoulder-width apart, and slowly begin to walk your hands down the back of the chair as you lift your chest up.

3. Keep your shoulders relaxed and your elbows slightly bent as you lift your chest and stretch your spine.

4. Hold the pose for a few deep breaths, allowing your breath to deepen the stretch.

5. To release the pose, slowly walk your hands back up the chair and come back to a seated position.

Here are a final few safety tips to keep in mind while performing your seated cobra sequence.

• Avoid overstretching your spine or forcing yourself deeper into the pose. Listen to your body and only go as far as feels comfortable.

• Keep your shoulders relaxed and your neck long to avoid any strain.

## Seated Half-Moon Pose

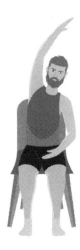

With this pose, you will be stretching your body while seated on a chair. It is a variation of the traditional Half Moon Pose, which is usually performed while you are standing up. It has been developed as a way to modify the traditional Half Moon Pose for those who may have difficulty standing for long periods.

This is how you're going to perform your pose:

1. Start off being seated on a chair with your feet flat on the floor and your hands resting on your thighs.

2. Place your right hand on the right side of the chair, just outside of your right hip.

3. Inhale and lift your left arm towards the ceiling, stretching it over your head and to the right side of your body.

4. Lean your torso to the right, stretching your left arm and side body as far as feels comfortable.

5. Hold the pose for a few deep breaths, feeling the stretch in the left side of your body.

6. Slowly come back to a seated position and repeat on the other side.

Some safety tips to keep in mind while performing the Seated Half Moon Pose:

• Keep your shoulders relaxed and your neck long throughout the pose.

• Do not overstretch your side body or force yourself deeper into the pose. Listen to your body and only go as far as feels comfortable.

## Seated Child's Pose

Seated child's pose is a gentle, forward folding posture done while seated on the floor or a chair. It provides a calming stretch for the back, shoulders, and hips. You do it by:

1. Sitting towards the front edge of your chair, feet flat on the floor about hip-width apart.

2. Exhale and fold your torso forward, walking your hands out towards the front of the chair.

3. Release your head and neck towards the floor or seat of the chair in front of you. Allow your shoulders to relax down your back.

4. You can keep your knees together or let them splay out wide for a deeper hip stretch.

5. Stay here, breathing deeply into the areas that feel tightest, for 5-10 breaths.

6. To release, slowly roll up one vertebra at a time with an inhale.

**Safety tips:**

- Don't force or bounce. Move gently and breathe deeply into areas of tension.

- Use a cushion or folded blanket under your knees if your hips are very tight.

- Don't strain your neck. Allow your head to hang heavy.

- If you have any injuries or concerns, you can do this pose while seated against a wall.

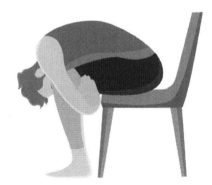

# Chapter Six

# Flexibility, Stability, and Balance Enhancing Chair Yoga Poses

My uncle was a very interesting man, he used to say, "You know, I'm not the supple leopard that I was in my youth." We would all laugh, but you could tell there was a hint of truth in his jest. As I watched him navigate the challenges of aging, I began to understand what he meant. I remember that there was a time when he could touch his toes with ease, his body bending and stretching with the same fluidity of a dancer, but as the years passed, I noticed a change. His movements became stiffer, his range of motion more limited; simple tasks like reaching for a high shelf or tying his shoes became arduous feats.

Despite his once-active lifestyle, the effects of aging were catching up with him. It wasn't just about losing physical capabilities; it was also about losing a sense of freedom and independence. The more his body stiffened, the more he withdrew from activities he once enjoyed.

One day, I found him sitting in his favorite chair, a wistful look in his eyes as he gazed out the window. "Getting old ain't for sissies," he remarked with a rueful smile. I sat beside him, feeling a pang of empathy for the changes he was experiencing. The more we talked, he shared his frustrations about the loss of flexibility that had crept up on him over the years. He spoke of the simple pleasures he missed—taking long walks without his joints protesting, playing with his grandchildren without worrying about pulling a muscle. It was a poignant moment that made me reflect on my own body and the inevitability of aging.

Watching him navigate the challenges of growing older, made me realize that flexibility is not just about physical mobility – it's also about adaptability, resilience, and the ability to embrace change. We lose flexibility in our bodies as we age, but we also lose it in our minds and spirits if we're not mindful. Flexibility is a precious gift, one that we must nurture and cherish throughout our lives. It's not about being the supple leopard of our youth, but about finding grace and strength in every stage of life. As I pondered his words, I knew that there was more to flexibility than meets the eye—and perhaps, in exploring the depths of this concept, I would discover a path to greater well-being and vitality.

## Regaining Stability and Flexibility

When we age, our bodies undergo various changes that affect how we once used to move here are some of the key reasons:

- **Loss of Muscle Mass:** As we age, we tend to lose muscle mass, a condition known as sarcopenia. This loss of muscle mass can lead to decreased strength and flexibility, making it harder to move and maintain balance.

- **Reduced Joint Flexibility:** Over time, the joints in our bodies may become stiffer due to wear and tear, decreased lubrication, and changes in the cartilage. This can limit our range of motion and contribute to decreased flexibility.

- **Changes in Connective Tissues**: The connective tissues in our bodies, such as tendons and ligaments, may become less elastic with age. This can affect joint mobility and stability, making movements feel more rigid and increasing the risk of injuries.

- **Decline in Bone Density**: Osteoporosis, a condition characterized by reduced bone density and strength, is common in older adults. Weak bones can make individuals more prone to fractures and impact their overall stability and confidence in movement.

- **Postural Changes:** As we age, changes in posture may occur due to factors such as muscle imbalances, decreased bone density, and reduced flexibility. Poor posture can lead to muscle tightness, discomfort, and an increased risk of falls.

- **Nervous System Changes:** The nervous system plays a crucial role in coordinating movement and maintaining balance. Age-related changes in nerve function and response time can impact muscle coordination and stability, affecting overall mobility.

- **Lifestyle Factors:** Sedentary lifestyles, lack of regular physical activity, and poor nutrition can also contribute to flexibility and stability issues as we age. Engaging in regular exercise, including activities that promote flexibility, strength, and balance, can help mitigate these effects.

## Seated Cactus Arms

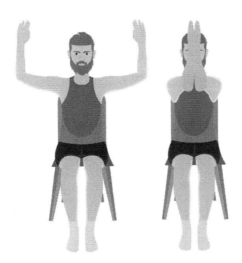

The seated cactus is a pose where you sit and bring your arms out to the side. You bend your knees at a 90-degree angle like a cactus to work your chest and shoulders. helps improve shoulder mobility and posture. Here is a detailed instruction on how you're going to perform seated cactus arms:

1. Sit tall in a sturdy chair with your feet flat on the ground, hip-width apart. Place your hands on your thighs or knees for support.

2. Take a moment to relax your shoulders down away from your ears, lengthening your spine.

3. Inhale as you lift your arms out to the sides at shoulder height, keeping your elbows bent at a 90-degree angle. Your forearms should be vertical, with your palms facing forward.

4. Imagine squeezing a ball between your shoulder blades to engage the muscles in your upper back.

5. Exhale as you gently draw your elbows back, opening up your chest and pulling your shoulder blades together. Feel a stretch across your chest and the front of your shoulders.

6. Hold the pose for 3-5 breaths, breathing deeply and maintaining a comfortable stretch. Keep your neck long and avoid shrugging your shoulders up towards your ears.

7. To release, inhale as you slowly bring your arms back to the starting position, lowering them down by your sides.

**Safety tips:**

- **Listen to your body**: If you feel any pain or discomfort in your shoulders or neck, ease out of the pose immediately.

- **Modify as needed**: If you have shoulder injuries or limited mobility, you can adjust the arm position to a comfortable range of motion that works for you.

- **Avoid locking your elbows**: Keep a slight bend in your elbows throughout the pose to prevent strain on the joints.

## Seated Palm Tree

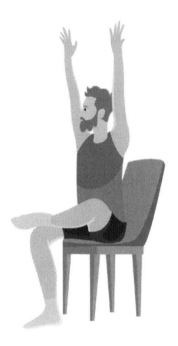

This is a seated pose that can be done in a chair and is similar to the Tree Pose in standing yoga. Here is how you perform the pose:

1. Start by sitting tall in a sturdy chair with your feet flat on the ground, hip-width apart. Place your hands on your knees or thighs for support.

2. Take a moment to relax your shoulders down away from your ears and lengthen your spine.

3. Slowly lift your right foot and place the sole of your right foot on your left inner thigh, with your toes pointing towards the floor.

4. Press your right foot into your left thigh to create a stable foundation.

5. Bring your hands in front of your heart, with your palms together in a prayer position.

6. On an inhale, raise your hands up above your head, keeping your palms together.

7. As you exhale, slowly lean to the left, keeping your hips rooted in the chair and your right foot pressing into your left thigh.

8. Take 3-5 deep breaths in this position, feeling a stretch through the right side of your body.

9. Inhale and return to an upright position with your hands in a prayer position.

10. Release your right foot back to the floor and repeat the pose on the other side.

**Safety tips:**

- If you have limited flexibility, you can modify the pose by placing your foot on your calf instead of your thigh.

- Maintain a stable foundation by keeping your hips rooted in the chair and avoiding leaning too far to the side.

- Keep your spine lengthened, so maintain an upright and aligned spine throughout the pose to support proper breathing and body alignment.

## Warrior II

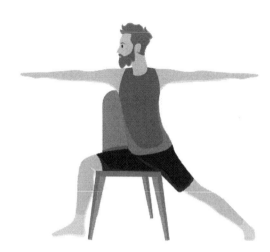

Warrior II is a modified version of the traditional Warrior II because it's done seated in a chair. It requires you to sit upright with one leg to the side and the other leg bent at a 90-degree angle while reaching your arms out to the side. Here's a step-by-step on how to complete the pose:

1. Start by sitting tall in a sturdy chair with your feet flat on the ground, hip-width apart. Place your hands on your knees or thighs for support.

2. Take a moment to relax your shoulders down away from your ears and lengthen your spine.

3. Slowly lift your right foot and place the sole of your right foot on your left inner thigh, with your toes pointing towards the floor.

4. Turn your torso to the right and bring your right knee towards your right shoulder.

5. Place your right hand on the outside of your right knee and reach your left arm up towards the ceiling.

6. As you exhale, slowly extend your right leg out to the side, keeping your right hand on your knee and your left arm reaching up towards the ceiling.

7. Gaze over your left shoulder and hold the pose for 3-5 deep breaths.

8. Inhale and return to an upright position with your hands on your knees or

thighs.

9. Release your right foot back to the floor and repeat the pose on the other side.

Here are some safety tips for consideration during the pose:

- If you have any knee or hip injuries, practice the pose with caution or avoid it altogether.

- If you have limited flexibility or balance, you can modify the pose by keeping your foot on the floor and only reaching your arm upwards.

- Do not push yourself beyond your limits and avoid any discomfort or strain in the pose.

## Standing Twists

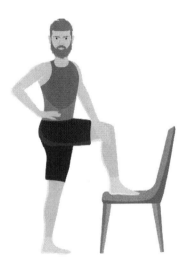

Standing twists involve twisting your torso while standing upright, which can help release tension and enhance your overall sense of well-being. This is how you carry them out:

1. Start by standing with your feet hip-width apart.

2. Place your hands on your hips and take a few deep breaths.

3. On an inhale, lift your right leg and place it on the chair in front of you.

4. Raise your arms up towards the ceiling and on an exhale, twist your torso to the right, bringing your left hand to your right hip and your right hand to the

small of your back.

5. Hold the pose for 3-5 deep breaths and then repeat on the other side.

These are some things you will need to remember as you do the pose:

- If you have any back, neck, or spine issues, practice the poses with caution or avoid them altogether.

- If you have limited flexibility or balance, you can modify the poses by keeping your hands on your hips or using an additional chair or wall for support.

- Do not push yourself beyond your limits and avoid any discomfort or strain in the poses. Focus on breathing deeply and moving slowly and mindfully.

## Ragdoll Pose

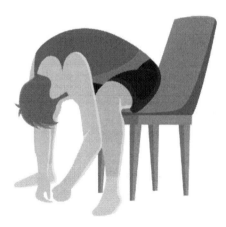

This is a forward fold that requires you to stand with your feet hip-width apart and bend forward at the hips while letting your torso hang loosely like a doll. It helps to release any tension you might have in the spine and hamstrings. This is how you do it:

1. Start by standing with your feet hip-width apart. Take a few deep breaths and allow your body to relax.

2. On an exhale, bend forward at the hips and let your head and arms hang down towards the floor. Allow your knees to bend as much as you need to in order to feel comfortable.

3. Hold onto opposite elbows with your hands and let your head and neck relax completely.

4. Take a few deep breaths and allow your body to release any tension.

5. If you would like to deepen the stretch, you can sway gently from side to side or shake your head yes and no.

6. Hold the pose for 30-60 seconds or longer if you would like.

7. To come out of the pose, slowly roll up one vertebrae at a time, allowing your head and neck to come up last.

As always, we value safety, so here are some things that you'll want to consider.

- If you have a history of back, neck, or spine issues, practice the pose with caution or avoid it altogether.

- If you have limited flexibility, you can modify the pose by using a chair or a wall for support. You can also keep your knees slightly bent if you feel any discomfort.

- Your body will give you cues to listen to. Do not push yourself beyond your limits and avoid any discomfort or strain in the pose. Focus on breathing deeply and releasing any tension in your body.

## Standing Half Split

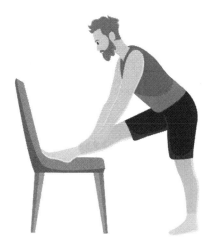

This is a pose that you're going to do standing, with one foot forward on the chair, and the other one on the floor. You will hinge at the hips to ring your torso parallel to the floor while flexing the front foot and extending the back leg straight behind you. Here are more instructions for performing the pose:

1. Start by standing with your feet hip-width apart. Take a few deep breaths and allow your body to relax.

2. Step your right foot forward and place it on the chair in front of you.

3. On an exhale, slowly straighten your right leg and hinge forward at the hips, placing your hands on your right thigh for support.

4. Allow your left leg to remain slightly bent and keep your left foot on the ground.

5. Flex your right foot and engage your quadriceps to protect your knee, if you require a deeper stretch.

6. Hold the pose for 3-5 deep breaths, feeling a stretch in your right hamstring.

7. Repeat the pose on the other side.

Here are some safety tips for you:

• Be extra cautious if you have any knee or hip injuries, practice the pose with caution or avoid it altogether.

• To protect your knee, engage your quadriceps and flex your right foot while performing the pose. This will help you maintain proper alignment and prevent any strain or injury.

## Chair Lunge

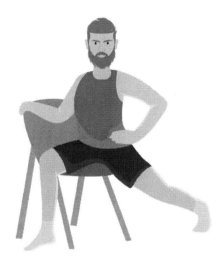

- Start by sitting tall in a sturdy chair with your feet flat on the ground, hip-width apart. Place your hands on your knees or thighs for support.

- Take a moment to relax your shoulders down away from your ears and lengthen your spine.

- Slowly lift your right foot and place the sole of your right foot on the floor, with your toes pointing towards the right side of the chair.

- Take a deep inhale and as you exhale, slide your left foot back, keeping your toes on the ground.

- Bend your right knee and sink down into a lunge position, keeping your left foot behind you.

- Keep your hands on your knees or thighs for support and hold the pose for 3-5 deep breaths.

- Alternatively, for a deeper lunge, place one hand on the back of the chair and one hand on your hip.

- Inhale and come back to a neutral position.

- Take a couple of breaths and repeat the exercise on the other side.

Here are some safety tips for performing the Chair Lunge:

- If you have issues with any knee or hip injuries, practice the pose with caution or avoid it altogether.

- If you have limited flexibility or balance, you can modify the pose by not sinking down as low into the lunge.

- Ensure that you maintain an upright and aligned spine throughout the pose to support proper breathing and body alignment.

# Chapter Seven

# Strength-Building Poses to Increase Muscle Mass

The truth is, while cardiovascular health is undeniably important for overall well-being, the role of strength training—especially as we age—should not be underestimated. Strength training is not just about building muscle for aesthetics; it's about maintaining the muscle mass that naturally diminishes as we grow older.

Let's take the story of Tom, a friend I've known for years. Tom was an avid runner, pounding the pavement day in and day out, believing that if he kept his heart strong and his weight down, he'd be the very picture of health. But as Tom crossed into his fifties, he noticed changes that his regular cardio routine didn't seem to address. His joints were sore, his posture had begun to stoop, and he felt a general weakness in performing everyday tasks that used to be second nature.

It wasn't until his doctor pointed out the importance of muscle mass for maintaining bone density, metabolic rate, and functional independence that he began to explore strength training. At first, he was skeptical. The weight room was a foreign world, filled with equipment that seemed intimidating and unnecessary for a man who had always prioritized heart rate over muscle tone.

But he took the plunge, and after several months of consistent, dedicated strength training, the differences were not just visible; they were palpable. His energy levels were up, his body felt firmer and more capable, and those everyday tasks? They were easier than they'd been in years. Tom learned that muscle mass isn't just for the young or the bodybuilders—it's for anyone who wants to live a full, active life at any age.

Strength training, it turns out, is not just about lifting weights; it's about lifting ourselves up to a higher standard of living as we age. It's about ensuring that our bodies continue to serve us, to carry us through the adventures we've yet to have. It is, in many ways, the foundation upon which a healthy, active lifestyle is built as we grow older.

So, as you explore the strength-building poses designed to increase muscle mass, remember this story. Remember that strength is not just about the external; it's about reinforcing the inner structures that support our very essence. And with each pose, we're not just moving; we're building a stronger, more resilient version of ourselves for the years to come.

## Building Strength and Muscle Mass With Chair Yoga

Slow controlled movements are vital for building strength and muscle mass. To understand the importance, let's liken it to running a marathon. You wouldn't sprint a marathon from start to finish because that would exhaust you quickly and increase the risk of injury. Similarly, slow and controlled movements in strength training allow for several key benefits:

- **Muscle Engagement**: When you perform exercises slowly and with control, your muscles are engaged throughout the entire range of motion. This ensures that you are targeting the specific muscle groups intended for that exercise, leading to more effective results.

- **Muscle Activation**: Moving slowly allows you to focus on the muscle being worked and ensures that it's doing the majority of the work, rather than relying on momentum or other assisting muscles. This targeted activation helps in building strength in the intended areas.

- **Muscle Fiber Recruitment**: Slow movements enable the recruitment of a higher number of muscle fibers. This is crucial for muscle growth and overall strength development. By moving slowly, you maximize the involvement of different muscle fibers, leading to better overall muscle mass gains.

- **Joint Stability**: Controlled movements reduce the risk of jerky, uncontrolled motions that can strain joints and connective tissues. Over time, this can help improve joint stability and reduce the likelihood of injuries, especially important for older individuals.

- **Mind-Muscle Connection**: Performing exercises slowly enhances the mind-muscle connection. You become more aware of the specific muscles being worked on and can focus on contracting them effectively, leading to better results and a deeper understanding of your body's movement patterns.

## Shoulder Press Using A Chair

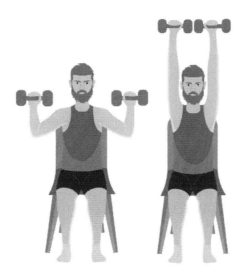

For the shoulder press exercise using a chair, here is a detailed step-by-step guide for your readers:

1. Begin by sitting tall on the edge of a sturdy chair with your feet flat on the floor, hip-width apart. Maintain good posture with your spine straight and shoulders relaxed.

2. Hold a weight (dumbbell or any suitable household item with some weight) in each hand at shoulder height. Your palms should be facing forward, and your elbows slightly in front of your shoulders.

3. Inhale and slowly press the weights upwards towards the ceiling, fully extending your arms without locking your elbows. Keep your core engaged to support your lower back.

4. As you exhale, slowly lower the weights back to the starting position at shoulder height. Focus on a smooth and controlled movement both on the way up and down.

5. Perform the shoulder press for the desired number of repetitions, maintaining proper form throughout. Aim for a pace that allows you to focus on muscle

engagement and control.

**Safety Tips:**

- Choose the right weights: Start with lighter weights to master the form before progressing to heavier weights. Using weights that are too heavy can strain your shoulders and lead to injury.

- Focus on stability: Maintain stable seating on the chair throughout the exercise. Avoid rocking back and forth or using momentum to lift the weights.

- Range of motion is important: Ensure you have a full range of motion during the shoulder press. Avoid going too low where your elbows drop below shoulder level, as this can strain the shoulder joint.

- Breathe: Remember to breathe throughout the exercise. Inhale as you prepare to lift the weights, and exhale as you press them upwards.

## Tricep Dips

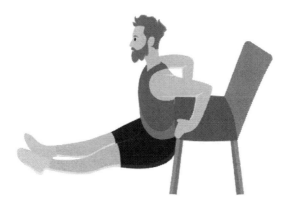

Tricep dips are a strength training exercise that targets the triceps muscles, which are located at the back of your upper arms. Always start with a lower number of reps and work your way up gradually. They can be quite challenging, so proper form is essential to avoid injury. Listen to your body and don't push through pain.

1. Sit on the floor with your legs extended in front of you.

2. Reach back and place your hands on the chair behind you, bend your elbows at 90 degrees, and make sure you have a proper grip.

3. Straighten your arms to lift your body off the floor, keeping your back close to

the chair.

4. Bend your elbows to lower your body toward the floor until your upper arms are parallel to the ground.

5. Straighten your arms to push yourself back up to the starting position.

6. Repeat

**Safety Tips**

- Keep your elbows tucked close to your body and pointed straight back, not flared out to the sides. This helps prevent strain on your elbow joints.

- Engage your core muscles to keep your body in a straight line from head to heels. Avoid arching your lower back or leaning too far forward.

- If the full exercise is too difficult, you can modify it by placing your feet flat on the floor in front of you, or by elevating your hands on a bench or chair.

## Chair Sun Salutation

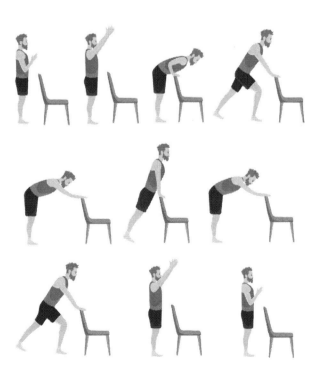

Chair Sun Salutations are a modified version of the traditional Sun Salutation (Surya Namaskar) sequence, performed using a chair for support and balance. This variation makes the practice more accessible for limited mobility, injury, or if you prefer a gentler form of exercise.

1. Begin by standing behind a sturdy chair, with your feet hip-width apart.

2. Inhale and raise your arms overhead, keeping your shoulders relaxed.

3. Exhale and fold forward from the hips, bringing your hands to the chair seat or the back of the chair, depending on your flexibility.

4. Inhale and lift your torso halfway up, creating a flat back and looking straight ahead.

5. Exhale and fold forward again, bringing your hands to the chair.

6. Inhale and lift your torso back to the standing position, raising your arms overhead.

7. Exhale and lower your arms to your sides.

You can repeat this several times, moving at a pace that suits your comfort level and breath. As you become more comfortable, you can incorporate additional movements, such as:

- Raising one leg back into a lunge position while keeping your hands on the chair for support.

- Twisting your torso from side to side while standing or in the forward fold position.

- Extending one leg out to the side, keeping your foot flat on the floor, for a gentle lateral stretch.

Some safety recommendations to keep in mind while practicing chair sun salutations include:

- Make sure your chair is stable and won't move around during your practice.

- Listen to your body and only move within your own range of motion. Do not force yourself into any position that causes pain.

- Always breathe deeply and slowly throughout your practice.

Remember to take your time with each movement and enjoy the benefits of chair sun salutations for your mind and body.

## Chair Sit-Ups

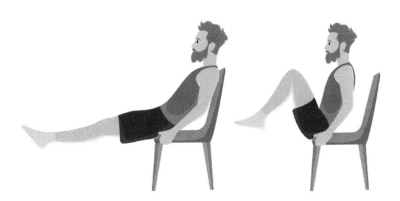

Chair situps are a great way to strengthen your core muscles and improve your overall fitness. They are easy to do and can be performed anywhere, making them perfect for men over 50 who want to stay active and healthy.

Here are the step-by-step instructions on how to perform chair situps:

1. Begin by sitting on the edge of your chair, with your feet flat on the ground and your hands placed on your thighs.

2. Inhale and lean back slightly, keeping your back straight and your core engaged.

3. Exhale and engage your abdominal muscles as you lift your feet off the ground and bring your knees towards your chest.

4. Inhale and slowly lower your feet back down to the ground.

5. Repeat this movement for 10-15 reps, moving with your breath.

Some safety recommendations to keep in mind while practicing chair situps include:

- Make sure your chair is stable and won't move around during your practice.

- Listen to your body and only move within your own range of motion. Do not force yourself into any position that causes pain.

- If you have any pre-existing medical conditions or injuries, consult with your doctor before beginning any new exercise routine.

- Always breathe deeply and slowly throughout your practice.

Remember to take your time with each movement and enjoy the benefits of chair situps for your core strength and overall fitness.

## Deep Chair Squats

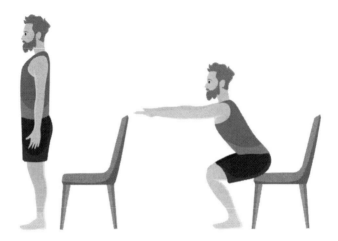

Deep chair squats are a modified version of the traditional squat exercise, designed to be performed while seated on a chair. This exercise is perfect for strengthening leg muscles and improving balance.

Here are the step-by-step instructions on how to perform deep chair squats:

1. Begin by sitting on the edge of your chair, with your feet planted firmly on the ground and your hands placed on your thighs.

2. Inhale and engage your core muscles as you stand up from the chair, keeping your back straight and your feet flat on the ground.

3. Exhale and slowly lower yourself back down into the chair, hovering just over the seat but not sitting down—keeping your knees bent and your core engaged.

4. Repeat this movement for 10-15 reps, moving with your breath.

Some safety recommendations to keep in mind while practicing deep chair squats include:

- Make sure your chair is stable and won't move around during your practice.

- Listen to your body and only move within your own range of motion. Do not force yourself into any position that causes pain.

Remember to take your time with each movement and enjoy the benefits.

## Advanced Chair Lunges

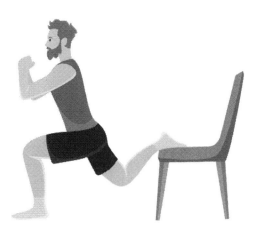

Advanced chair lunges are a challenging exercise that can help strengthen your leg muscles and improve your overall fitness. They are a modified version of the traditional lunge exercise, designed to be performed while holding onto the back of a chair for balance.

This is how you do them:

1. Stand with your back to a chair, with your feet hip-width apart and your hands at your sides.

2. Make sure your chair is backed against a wall so it won't move.

3. Inhale and place your left foot back on the chair.

4. Inhale and take a step forward with your right foot, lowering yourself into a lunge position.

5. Your right knee should be bent at a 90-degree angle.

6. Exhale and push off your right foot, returning to your starting position.

7. Repeat this movement with your left foot, taking a step forward and lowering yourself into a lunge position.

8. Repeat this sequence for 10-15 reps on each leg, moving with your breath.

9. If you cannot maintain balance, flip your chair around and use the backrest as support as you complete regular, standing lunges.

Some safety recommendations to keep in mind while practicing advanced chair lunges include:

• Make sure your chair is stable and won't move around during your practice.

• Listen to your body and only move within your own range of motion. Do not force yourself into any position that causes pain.

• If you have any pre-existing medical conditions or injuries, consult with your doctor

## Seated March

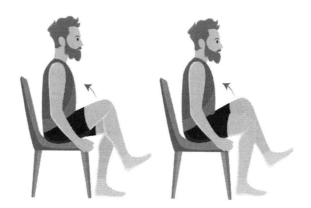

The seated march is an exercise where you mimic the motion of marching while seated. It involves lifting your knees one at a time towards your chest, engaging your core and lower body muscles. Remember that you can perform this at various speeds, this is what makes it suitable for beginner levels.

To perform the seated march:

1. Sit upright in a chair or on the floor with your back straight and abdominal muscles engaged.

2. Lift one knee towards your chest, keeping the other foot flat on the floor.

3. Alternate, lifting the opposite knee towards your chest while lowering the first

leg back down.

4. Continue alternating the marching motion, lifting your knees as high as comfortable and maintaining a steady rhythm.

Three safety tips for the seated march:

- Keep your core engaged and avoid arching your back or leaning backward as you lift each knee. Maintain an upright posture throughout the exercise.

- If you have knee or hip issues, avoid lifting your knees too high. Keep the range of motion comfortable and controlled.

- Breathe naturally throughout the exercise, avoiding holding your breath.

## Chapter Eight

# Heart Health–Specialized Chair Yoga Series

Heartbeats, I like to believe, are our bodies' languages of choice. Think about it, there are thousands of wordless signals passed through the skin. Moment by moment, orchestrating the symphony of life within us. Each beat represents a story, a journey, and a choice. As we age, these choices accumulate, shaping the health of our hearts and the quality of our lives. This truth became vividly clear to me one afternoon, as I sat in a cozy community center, surrounded by a group of seniors eager to explore the benefits of chair yoga for heart health.

The room was filled with a sense of anticipation and curiosity. I guided the class through a gentle warm-up, encouraging everyone to connect with their breath and set an intention for our practice. Among the participants was a sprightly woman in her late 70s, with a twinkle in her eye and a spring in her step that belied her age. She had been attending the chair yoga sessions regularly, eager to learn new ways to care for her heart and nurture her well-being.

As we moved through the poses, her dedication and enthusiasm were palpable. Her commitment to her practice was inspiring, as she gracefully navigated each movement with a sense of grace and determination. I couldn't help but marvel at her resilience and zest for life, embodying the belief that age is just a number, and that true vitality comes from within.

During a moment of rest, she shared with the rest of us a glimpse of her journey towards embracing a heart-healthy lifestyle. She spoke of a time when she had neglected her well-being, succumbing to the pressures of a fast-paced career and a sedentary lifestyle. It was a wake-up call—a health scare that shook her to the core and forced her to reevaluate her choices. She leaned towards healthier eating habits, prioritized regular physical activity, and sought out holistic practices like yoga to nourish her body, mind, and spirit. Through dedication and perseverance, she not only improved her physical health but also cultivated a deep sense of inner peace and resilience.

As I listened to her story, it really dawned on me; Her journey was a reminder of the importance of self-care in shaping our well-being as we age. It was a reminder that each heartbeat is a reflection of the choices we make—a silent language that speaks volumes about our commitment to health and vitality.

At that moment, surrounded by a community of kindred spirits on a shared journey towards better heart health, I felt a deep sense of gratitude for the opportunity to see such change radiate through the human spirit. Her story lit a spark within me, reminding me of the profound connection between our choices, our hearts, and our journey toward wellness.

## Heart Healthy Chair Yoga Poses

Heart healthy chair yoga poses are specifically designed to improve cardiovascular function, increase circulation, and strengthen the muscles surrounding the heart. When you incorporate these into your routine, you can take an active role in maintaining a healthy heart, all from the comfort and stability of a chair.

### Seated Warrior I

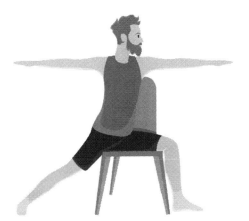

Seated Warrior I is a modified yoga pose that can be practiced in a chair and offers a gentle way to stretch and strengthen the body, particularly focusing on the legs, hips, and core muscles. This pose helps improve posture, balance, and stability while also encouraging a sense of grounding and strength.

Here is a detailed instruction for you on how you're going to perform the exercise

1. Start by sitting tall in a sturdy chair with your feet flat on the ground, hip-width apart.

2. Engage your core muscles and lengthen your spine as you take a deep breath in.

3. On an exhale, extend your right leg straight out in front of you, keeping your foot flexed and toes pointing up.

4. Inhale as you bend your left knee, bringing the foot back towards the chair, ensuring it is firmly planted on the ground.

5. Extend both arms toward your sides, reaching your fingers out to either side of you while keeping your shoulders relaxed.

6. Hold this position for a few breaths, feeling a gentle stretch in the front of your right hip and thigh.

7. To release, slowly lower your arms and return your right foot to the floor, coming back to the starting position.

## Safety Tips

- If you have any hip, knee, or back injuries, consult with a healthcare provider or a qualified yoga instructor before attempting this pose.

- Maintain proper alignment by keeping your spine lengthened and your core engaged throughout the pose.

- Use the chair for support and stability as needed, especially if you have balance issues or feel unsteady in the pose.

## Chair Eagle Pose

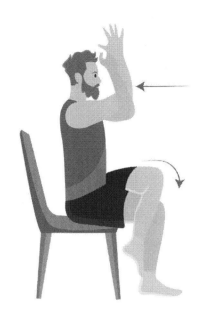

Chair eagle pose is a seated variation of the eagle pose and it involves you wrapping one leg around the other and crossing one arm underneath the other with the palms touching. It improves your balance, your focus, and your flexibility.

Here are the instructions on how to perform the chair eagle pose:

1. You're going to start seated, with your feet planted firmly on the ground and your spine straight.

2. Inhale and lift your right leg, crossing it over your left thigh. If possible, hook your right foot behind your left calf.

3. Inhale and lift your arms out to the sides, bringing them to shoulder height with your palms facing down.

4. Exhale and cross your left arm over your right arm, bending your elbows and bringing your palms to touch.

5. Hold this position for 5-10 deep breaths, focusing on your balance and concentration.

6. Release the pose and repeat on the other side.

## Safety Tips

- If you have knee or hip injuries, it is important to be cautious when crossing your legs and to avoid this pose if it causes any discomfort.

- If you have shoulder injuries or limited mobility in your arms, you can modify this pose by simply crossing your legs and bringing your hands to your heart center.

- Always listen to your body and move within your own range of motion. Do not force yourself into any position that causes pain or discomfort.

## Standing Half-Moon

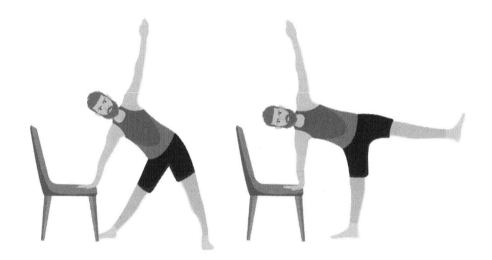

The standing half-moon, also known as Ardha Chandrasana in Sanskrit, is a popular yoga posture that helps to improve balance, strengthen the legs and core, and increase flexibility. It is a standing pose that requires a bit of focus and stability because you have to balance on one leg while extending the other leg and reaching the opposite arm out toward the sky.

This is how you perform the pose:

1. Begin in Mountain Pose, standing with your feet together and your arms at your sides.

2. Inhale and lift your arms above your head, reaching towards the ceiling.

3. Exhale and slowly bend to the right, sliding your left hand down your left leg

and reaching your right arm up towards the ceiling.

4. Keep your gaze towards your right hand and hold the pose for a few breaths.

5. Inhale and lift back up to the center, reaching your arms towards the ceiling.

6. Exhale and repeat on the left side, sliding your right hand down your right leg and reaching your left arm up towards the ceiling.

7. Hold the pose for a few breaths before returning to the center.

Some **safety recommendations** to keep in mind:

- If you have had any injuries, consult with your doctor before beginning any new exercise routine.

- Only move within your own range of motion. Do not force yourself into any position that causes pain.

- If you feel dizzy or lightheaded, come out of the pose slowly and take a few deep breaths before continuing.

Remember to take your time with each movement and enjoy the benefits

## Standing Tree Pose

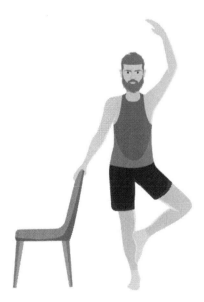

Standing Tree Pose, also known as Vrksasana in Sanskrit, is a popular yoga posture that helps to improve balance, focus, and flexibility. It requires you to stand on one leg with the sole of your other foot resting on your inner thigh or calf, with your hands in prayer position at your heart center.

This is how you will perform the pose:

1. Begin in Mountain Pose, standing with your feet together and your arms at your sides.

2. Shift your weight onto your left foot and lift your right foot off the ground, placing the sole of your right foot onto your left thigh. Keep your toes pointing towards the floor and your knee pointing out to the side.

3. Bring your hands together at your heart center and hold the pose for a few breaths.

4. If you feel stable, you can try lifting your arms above your head, reaching towards the ceiling.

5. Hold the pose for a few breaths before returning to Mountain Pose and repeating on the other side.

6. If you're not stable on your feet, use the back of your chair to maintain your balance.

Some safety recommendations to keep in mind:

- Listen to your body and only move within your own range of motion. Do not force yourself into any position that causes pain.

- If you feel dizzy or lightheaded, come out of the pose slowly and take a few deep breaths before continuing.

- If you have trouble balancing, you can place your foot on your ankle or calf instead of your thigh.

## Triangle Pose

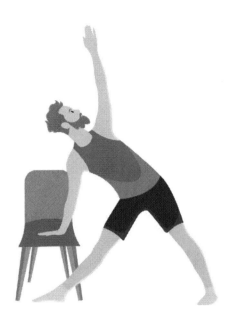

Triangle pose, also known as Trikonasana in Sanskrit, is a popular yoga posture that helps to stretch the legs, hips, and spine, and improve balance and stability. It is a standing pose that requires a bit of focus and flexibility, making it a great addition to any yoga practice.

Here is your detailed step-by-step guide:

1. Begin in Mountain Pose, standing with your feet together and your arms at your sides.

2. Step your feet about 3-4 feet apart, with your toes pointing forward.

3. Turn your right foot out 90 degrees and your left foot in slightly.

4. Inhale and lift your arms to shoulder height, keeping them parallel to the floor.

5. Exhale and reach your right arm forward, tilting your torso to the right and bringing your right hand down to your chair.

6. Extend your left arm towards the ceiling, keeping your gaze towards your left hand.

7. Hold the pose for a few breaths before returning to the center and repeating on the other side.

Some safety recommendations to keep in mind:

- Do not force yourself into any position that causes pain.

- Keep your knee straight but not locked. If you have knee pain, you can bend your knee slightly.

- If you feel dizzy or lightheaded, come out of the pose slowly and take a few deep breaths before continuing.

## Half-Sun Salutation

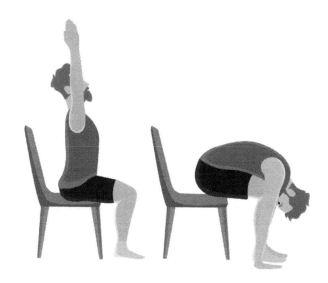

Half Sun Salutation is a modified version of the traditional Sun Salutation sequence that is designed to be performed while sitting on a chair. It typically involves you moving from mountain pose to your forward fold, then to a halfway lift, and then back to mountain pose. It is a great way for you to loosen up your joints, stretch your muscles, and energize your body.

Here are the step-by-step instructions on how to perform Half Sun Salutation in chair yoga:

1. Begin in a comfortable seated position, with your feet planted firmly on the ground and your spine straight.

2. Inhale and raise your arms above your head, reaching towards the ceiling.

3. Exhale and bring your hands down to your heart center.

4. Inhale lean forward so that your hands touch your ankles, if possible.

5. Exhale and lift your body up, hinging at the hips but remaining seated.

6. Inhale and lift your arms again, reaching towards the ceiling.

7. Exhale and bring your hands back down to your sides.

You can repeat this sequence for 5-10 rounds, moving with your breath.

Some **safety recommendations** to keep in mind during your practice:

- Make sure your chair is stable and won't move around during your practice.

- Always breathe deeply and slowly throughout your practice.

Remember to take your time with each movement and enjoy the benefits of the pose. It's a great way to energize and loosen your body in a gentle and safe way.

## Single Leg Forward Bend

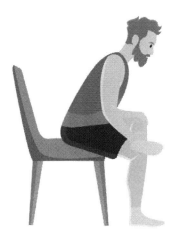

This is a pose that helps to stretch the hamstrings, calves, and hips, and improve balance and flexibility. You sit with one of your legs extended straight in front of you and then fold forward over the extended leg, reaching toward your toes. Here are the step-by-step instructions:

1. Position yourself comfortably in your chair, with your feet planted firmly on the ground and your spine straight.

2. Lift your right foot off the ground and place the sole of your foot onto your left

inner thigh. Keep your toes pointing towards the floor and your knee pointing out to the side.

3. Exhale and hinge forward at the hips, keeping your back straight and your gaze towards the ground.

4. Reach your hands towards your left foot, keeping your left knee bent.

5. Hold the pose for a few breaths before returning to a seated position and repeating on the other side.

Things to keep in mind as you practice:

- Make sure your chair is stable and won't move around during your practice.

- Keep your knee straight but not locked. If you have knee pain, you can bend your knee slightly.

# Chapter Nine

# Cooling Down—Relaxation Poses

R emember how I told you that I practically never warmed up before exercising, while I never really cooled down as well? It was a habit born out of impatience and a desire to maximize every minute of my workout. For years, I would dive headfirst into intense physical activity, pushing my body to its limits without giving much thought to the importance of a proper cool-down.

Little did I know, I was doing my body a great disservice by skipping this crucial step. Without a gradual transition to rest, my muscles would remain tense and contracted, depriving them of the oxygen-rich blood flow needed for recovery. The lactic acid buildup would linger, leaving me feeling stiff and sore for days after. My mind, still buzzing with adrenaline, would struggle to find the calm and clarity I so desperately craved after exerting myself.

It wasn't until I discovered the profound benefits of cooling down that I realized how essential it is to treat this phase with the same reverence as the warmup and main workout. A proper cool down allows the body to ease back into its resting state, promoting flexibility, accelerating muscle repair, and quieting the mind's flurry of activity. It's the gentle Landing that prevents the jarring impact of an abrupt halt, setting the stage for renewed energy and vitality on your next journey into movement.

## Cooling Down

Even if you don't feel tired, it is essential to incorporate a proper cool down into your exercise routine. Cooling down is not just about addressing fatigue; it plays a crucial role in allowing the body to transition from a state of exertion to a state of rest, promoting recovery and reducing the risk of injury.

Muscle stiffness can occur for various reasons, one of which is the accumulation of waste products such as lactic acid in the muscles during intense physical activity. Without a proper cool-down, these waste products can linger in the muscles, contributing to soreness, stiffness, and decreased flexibility. Cooling down helps facilitate the removal of these waste products by promoting blood flow and lymphatic drainage, aiding in the body's natural recovery process.

Furthermore, when we exercise, our muscles contract and shorten, leading to increased muscle tension. If we abruptly stop physical activity without allowing our muscles to gradually return to their resting length, it can result in muscle tightness and discomfort. Cooling down with gentle stretches and movements helps elongate the muscles, releasing tension and promoting flexibility.

Additionally, cooling down allows the heart rate and breathing rate to gradually return to baseline levels, preventing a sudden drop in blood pressure that can lead to dizziness or fainting. It also helps regulate body temperature, preventing a rapid cooling that can occur if we stop moving abruptly after a workout.

Incorporating a proper cool down into your exercise routine, even when you don't feel tired, is essential for maintaining overall physical well-being and optimizing the benefits of your workout. By taking the time to cool down with gentle stretching, deep breathing, and relaxation techniques, you can support your body's recovery process, reduce muscle stiffness, and promote long-term fitness and health. Remember, caring for your body after exercise is just as important as the effort you put into your workout.

## Seated Happy Baby Pose

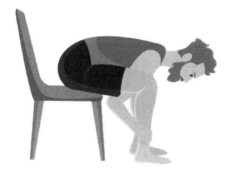

Seated Baby Pose is a gentle yoga pose that can help to relax the body and calm the mind. It is a variation of Child's Pose, typically performed in a seated position instead of on hands and knees. This pose is great for stretching the back, hips, and thighs, and it can help release tension in the lower back.

Here's how you can do it:

1. Sit on a chair with your feet flat on the floor, hip-width apart.

2. Slowly lower your torso forward, allowing your chest to rest on or between your thighs.

3. Extend your arms forward on the chair or reach for the floor in front of the chair, whichever is more comfortable for you.

4. Relax your forehead on the chair seat or let it hang freely.

5. Take slow, deep breaths and relax in this position for 1-2 minutes, feeling the gentle stretch in your back, hips, and thighs.

## Seated Five-Point Star

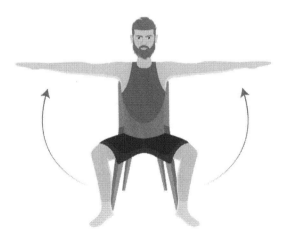

The Seated Five-Point Star is a chair yoga pose that helps to open up the chest, shoulders, and upper back while also engaging the core muscles. Here's how to do it:

1. Sit towards the front edge of your chair, keeping your feet flat on the floor and your spine straight.

2. Extend your right arm out to the side, parallel to the floor, forming one "point" of the star.

3. Extend your left leg out to the side, keeping your foot flexed and forming another "point" of the star.

4. Reach your left arm up towards the ceiling, forming the third point.

5. Extend your right leg out to the side, keeping your foot flexed and forming the fourth point.

6. Gently twist your upper body to the right, allowing your gaze to follow your right hand behind you, forming the fifth and final point of the star.

7. Hold this position for a few deep breaths, feeling the stretch across your chest, shoulders, and back.

8. Slowly release and repeat on the opposite side.

When performing the Seated Five-Point Star, remember to:

- Keep your abdominal muscles engaged to support your spine and prevent arching your back.

- Avoid straining or forcing the stretch. Move within a comfortable range of motion.

- Use the chair for support if needed, placing your hands on the seat or armrests to maintain balance.

## Puppy Dog Pose

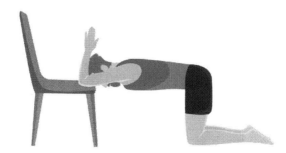

The Puppy Dog Pose (Uttana Shishosana) is a gentle backbend that stretches the spine, shoulders, and hip flexors. This pose is a gentle way to stretch the spine, open the shoulders, and release tension in the back and hips. It can be a great counter-pose after sitting for extended periods or forward-folding poses. Here's how to perform this pose:

1. Start on your hands and knees, with your hands on the seating area of your chair.

2. Walk your hands forward, keeping your arms extended and your hips over your knees.

3. Allow your chest to sink towards the chair as you slide.

4. Rest your forehead on the chair, and relax your neck.

5. Bend your elbows to 90 degrees and bring your palms together at the back of your head.

6. Engage your core and slightly tuck your tailbone under to maintain the backbend.

7. Breathe deeply and hold the pose for several breaths.

8. To release, walk your hands back towards your body and return to a neutral tabletop position.

When practicing puppy dog pose, keep these tips in mind:

- Go slowly and don't force the backbend. Only extend as far as is comfortable for your body.

- Keep your core engaged to protect your lower back from excessive arching.

- If you feel any strain or discomfort in your neck, place a cushion or folded blanket under your forehead for support.

## Chair Bridge

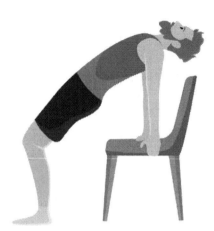

The Chair Bridge Pose is a gentle backbend that can be performed while seated in a chair. It can help improve spinal mobility, open up the chest and shoulders, and strengthen the muscles in the back, glutes, and hamstring: Here's how to do it:

1. Sit towards the front edge of the chair, with your feet flat on the floor, hip-width apart.

2. Place your hands on the chair beside your hips, fingers pointing toward the back of the chair.

3. Inhale and lift your hips off the chair, creating a straight line from your knees to your shoulders.

4. Gently engage your core muscles and avoid arching your lower back excessively.

5. If comfortable, you can clasp your hands behind your back and lift your chest towards the ceiling.

6. Keep your gaze forward or slightly upward, being mindful not to strain your neck.

7. Hold the pose for several breaths, focusing on your breathing and engaging your glutes and hamstrings.

8. Exhale and slowly lower your hips back down to the chair seat.

Three important tips to remember:

- Use your arm strength to support your body weight and avoid putting too much pressure on your neck or shoulders.

- If you have limited mobility or tightness in your hips or back, keep the backbend gentle and don't overarch.

- Engage your core muscles throughout the pose to protect your lower back.

# Chapter Ten

# Nutritional Support–Building Your Body From the Inside Out

Y ou cannot claim to love your body and then not nourish it in the way that it deserves to be nourished. And by nourishment, I am not saying deny yourself of your favorite foods. By nourish, I mean you feed it well and you give it what it loves occasionally too, something like a gooey, sticky brownie, complete with a glass of cold milk to wash it down.

As men, we often neglect our nutritional needs, especially as we get older. We justify greasy food, an extra beer, or skipping meals entirely with a casual "I'm a guy, it doesn't matter." But it does matter, especially if you are engaging in physical activity like the chair yoga routines in this book.

Proper nutrition is the foundation for an energized, lean, and healthy body at any age. You can't build a sturdy house without a solid foundation, and you can't build an energized, capable body without feeding it the right stuff. Think of nutrition as the bricks and mortar that build and maintain your body's capacity for movement, strength, and vitality.

And just like constructing a house, you need a consistent supply of quality materials—in this case, a balanced diet of protein, healthy fats, complex carbs, vitamins, and minerals. Skimp on any of those and your body's physical performance and stamina will suffer. Your muscles won't recover well from the yogic stretches and poses. Your energy levels will plummet by mid-afternoon. You'll feel achy, sluggish, and less able to embrace all life has to offer.

So consider this chapter your nutrition blueprint. Follow it and you'll uphold your end of the deal with your body—giving it the nutritious fuel it needs to sustain you through the chair yoga practice and beyond. You'll rediscover vitality, alertness, and a trimmer waistline too. And you can still indulge in your favorite treats on occasion, like that gooey brownie. After all, what's life without a little sweetness?

## Nutrition for Senior Men

Your body is no longer what it was when you were 16, or 21, or even 30, so that naturally then means that your nutritional needs are going to be different. Let's take a look at the key shifts that happen in your body as you age:

- Your metabolism tends to slow down as you get older, meaning you'll burn fewer calories than you did in your youth. This makes weight management trickier and makes it even more important to eat a nutrient-dense diet full of foods that provide lasting energy, not empty calories.

- Muscle mass also tends to decline with age if you don't take steps to preserve it. Getting adequate protein becomes crucial for maintaining and building strength. Seniors need about 0.5-0.6 grams of protein per pound of body weight to prevent muscle wasting.

- Calcium, vitamin D, magnesium, and other bone-supporting nutrients are essential for preventing osteoporosis and bone fractures as testosterone levels drop. Dairy, leafy greens, fatty fish, and proper sun exposure can help optimize bone density.

- Many men over 50 are managing conditions like high blood pressure, high cholesterol, diabetes, or arthritis through diet and lifestyle changes. The right nutritional intake of sodium, fiber, healthy fats, and anti-inflammatory foods becomes very important.

- Staying properly hydrated gets tougher as you age and your thirst signals aren't as strong. Proper fluid intake supports energy levels, digestion, cognitive function, and more. Aim for at least 64 oz of water daily.

The physical demands of chair yoga along with the natural aging process mean your body's nutritional needs will shift as well, so paying close attention to getting the right nutrients becomes key to supporting your health, energy, and active lifestyle.

## *Understanding Macronutrients*

I'm sure you've heard of the term "macronutrient" somewhere between now and a long time ago, but let's quickly recap what it means. Macronutrients are the three main categories of nutrients you need in relatively large amounts to provide energy, growth, and other bodily functions—carbohydrates, proteins, and fats.

Carbohydrates are your body's preferred source of fuel, especially for your brain and active muscles during yoga. Emphasize complex carbs like whole grains, fruits, veggies, and legumes over simple sugars.

Protein provides the building blocks for repairing and maintaining lean muscle mass, which naturally declines with age. Good protein sources include lean meats, poultry, fish, eggs, dairy, nuts, and legumes.

Healthy fats are essential for nutrient absorption, brain health, hormone production, and regulating inflammation. Focus on unsaturated fats from plants, fatty fish, nuts, and olive oil.

While macros are crucial, micronutrients (vitamins and minerals) are like spark plugs allowing all the amazing biochemical reactions to fire properly. Key micronutrients for men over 50 include:

- Calcium and vitamin D for bone strength

- Magnesium for muscle and nerve function

- B vitamins for energy production

- Antioxidants like vitamins C and E to protect cells

- Zinc for immune function and wound healing

Even if you hit your macronutrient targets, not getting adequate micronutrients can lead to nutrient deficiencies, increased disease risk, and lack of vitality. This is why a balanced, whole food-based diet full of colorful fruits and veggies is so important as you age. It provides steady streams of the micro and macronutrients your body craves for robust health and an active chair yoga lifestyle.

## *Tips for Optimizing Nutrition*

Optimizing your nutrition doesn't have to be hard or all that complicated for that matter. Here are some simple tips to help you get the nutrients your body needs as an active man.

- **Plan properly**: Take 30 minutes on the weekend to plan out meals and snacks for the upcoming week. Having a plan makes it easier to shop for nutritious ingredients and prevents last-minute fast food detours.

- **Eat the rainbow:** Aim to get a variety of naturally colorful fruits and veggies on your plate at each meal. The more colors, the better the nutritional variety of vitamins, minerals, and antioxidants.

- **Prioritize protein**: Include a quality protein source like fish, lean meat, eggs, beans, or dairy at every meal. Adequate protein becomes even more crucial for maintaining muscle mass and strength as you age.

- **Drink your H2O**: Carry a reusable water bottle and sip regularly throughout the day. Proper hydration supports energy levels, focus, digestion, and recovery from your yoga practice.

- **Choose healthy fats**: Get a daily serving or two of healthy unsaturated fats from foods like salmon, avocados, olive oil, nuts, and seeds for heart, brain, and joint benefits.

- **Don't overcomplicate things**: Eating nutritiously doesn't require fancy supplements, pricey "superfoods," or complicated recipes. Focus on simple, wholesome ingredients prepared in an uncomplicated way.

- **Be mindful**: Check in with your hunger/fullness cues and eat mindfully without distractions. This ensures you meet your needs without overeating.

With these tips, you can create lasting nutrition habits to energize you through your chair yoga journey and all the adventures of life right now.

## *Key Lifestyle Considerations*

Nothing changes if nothing changes - it's as simple as that. While focusing on sound nutrition is crucial, there are other key lifestyle factors to consider for optimal health and vitality:

- **Exercise**. Chair yoga is excellent for flexibility, balance, and mobility, but also incorporates strength training to maintain muscle mass and bone density. Aim for 2-3 sessions per week focusing on all major muscle groups.

- **Sleep**. Prioritize getting 7-9 hours of quality sleep nightly. Poor sleep impacts everything from recovery and appetite regulation to cognitive function and disease risk. Establish a relaxing pre-bed routine.

- **Stress Management**. Chronic stress takes a massive toll on mental and physical health over time. Build regular stress relief into your routine through yoga, meditation, deep breathing, or other mindfulness practices.

- **Social Connection**. An active social life provides mental stimulation and emotional support, both of which contribute to overall well-being. Prioritize regular time with friends, family, clubs, or community groups.

- **Purpose & Passion**. Those things that leave a twinkle in your eye, things that give you meaning keep your mind sharp and give you drive. Don't stop living there's still so much more to life that you can leverage.

When your nutrition AND other pillars of a healthy lifestyle are addressed, you'll ensure you have the energy, strength, and vitality to make the most of these enriching years. Small, consistent changes compounded over time lead to powerful results.

I think I said it somewhere in this book, but you aren't a passive observer in your life. You aren't the supporting role in someone else's story. This is your life and you are the leading actor on the stage. The choices you make—what you eat, how you move, how you spend your time—those choices sculpt your daily experience and long-term well-being.

When you take hold of the reins and choose to optimize your nutrition and overall lifestyle, you are taking control of your health journey. You are choosing to build your physical resilience from the inside out through nutrient-dense foods. You are choosing to strengthen your bones and muscles through exercise. You are choosing to protect your cognitive vitality by managing stress.

These aren't passive choices, but powerful acts of self-care that shape your capabilities and independence as you age. The man who conquers the latest chair yoga routine with ease? The one who brings vibrant energy and an engaged mind to every conversation? That could be you if you fully commit to upholding your body's needs for nutritional support.

Don't live your life out on the sidelines. Nourish and strengthen yourself through your daily choices. Take center stage and play the leading role of a man who intends to live this season of life boldly and abundantly. The curtain is up—it's time to take your place in the spotlight.

## Chapter Eleven

# 28-Day Chair Yoga Challenge

They say that it takes approximately 20-30 days to develop a habit. Sounds like a very long time, doesn't it? But those days pass quickly when you are doing something enjoyable that makes you feel better. That's exactly what this 28-day chair yoga challenge is designed to do for you.

Over the next 4 weeks, you will be guided through a series of gentle yoga poses and breathing exercises, all performed from the comfort of a chair. Each day's routine builds upon the previous day, allowing you to incrementally advance your practice at a manageable pace. By the end of the 28 days, you'll have learned the essentials of chair yoga and developed a sustainable habit to continue long after the challenge is over.

The benefits of sticking with this challenge are numerous. You will improve your flexibility, balance, strength, and posture—areas that tend to decline as you get older. It's an empowering way to relieve tension, increase energy levels, and reduce stress and anxiety. Best of all, it can be done by anyone regardless of age, weight, or fitness level.

Beyond the physical perks, chair yoga encourages mindfulness through its emphasis on controlled breathing and being present in the moment. This mindfulness component can improve your focus, mood, and overall well-being. Many committed practitioners find chair yoga provides a sense of calmness they can draw upon no matter what life throws their way.

So open your mind to the benefits of this challenge. Follow along diligently for the next 28 days, believe me, your future self will thank you for the gift of increased strength, flexibility, and peace of mind. Let's get started!

# Your 28-Day Chair Yoga Challenge

Before starting, remember that you can do the warm-up exercises as we've explained in the previous chapters.

## *Week 1: Fundamental Chair Yoga Poses*

**Day 1:**

- Warm up with 5 minutes of neck rolls, arm circles, and shoulder shrugs.

- Practice mountain pose, cat/cow pose, and forward fold—holding each 5 breaths.

- Cool down with 5 minutes of seated meditation.

**Day 2:**

- Warm-up with gentle torso twists.

- Practice mountain pose with arms raised, seated backbend, and seated side stretch—8 breaths per pose.

- Cool down with seated baby pose.

**Day 3:**

- Warm up with shoulder rolls.

- Move through mountain pose, cat/cow, forward fold, and seated side bend - 5 breaths each.

- Cool down with a chair bridge pose stretch.

**Day 4:**

- Warm up with ankle rolls.

- Practice seated backbend, twist, and bound angle pose—8 breaths per pose.

- Cool down with grip strength exercise using a hand towel.

**Day 5:**

- Warm up with head circles.

- Move slowly through the seated mountain, cat/cow, and forward fold.

- Hold each 10 breaths. Cool down with alternate nostril breathing.

## *Week 2: Targeting Back Pain and Stiffness*

**Day 6:**

- Warm up with seated side stretch.

- Perform seated backbend, double leg stretch, and seated side bend—10 breaths each to relieve back tension.

- Cool down with wrist circles.

**Day 7:**

- Warm up with arm circles.

- Practice chair child's pose, seated forward fold, and seated twist—holding each 8-10 breaths to release lower back.

- Cool down with deep breathing.

**Day 8:**

- Warm up with neck rolls.

- Perform seated cat/cow, seated side stretch, and chair push-ups - 10 reps each to mobilize the upper back.

- Cool down with your shoulder rolls

**Day 9:**

- Warm-up with ankle rotations.

- Move through seated backbend, and seated cat-cow - 10 breaths each for lower back mobility.

- Cool down with meditation.

**Day 10:**

Rest Day

## *Week 3: Flexibility, Stability, and Balance*

**Day 11:**

- Warm up with seated cat cow pose.

- Start with knee to chest pose–10 breaths per side, then your seated chair pose, and end off with seated cobra pose. Repeat this flow 2 to 3 times before cooling down.

- Cool down with shoulder shrugs.

**Day 12:**

- Warm up with wrist circles.

- Hold seated forward fold, and seated twist—8-10 breaths per pose for hip and back flexibility.

- Cool down with shoulder shrugs.

**Day 13:**

- Warm up with gentle seated backbends.

- Move slowly through the seated mountain pose, chair knee raises, and heel raises —10 reps each for balance and stability.

- Cool down with deep breathing.

**Day 14:**

- Warm up with arm raises.

- Practice chair tree pose, chair warrior III, and chair leg raises—8 breaths per pose to improve balance and core strength.

- Cool down with neck stretches.

**Day 15:**

- Warm up with shoulder shrugs.

- Hold seated mountain pose, chair knee raises with arm extensions, and heel raises—10 breaths each for balance training.

- Cool down with meditation.

**Day 16:**

- Warm up with wrist and ankle rolls.

- Practice seated cactus arms, and ragdoll pose—10 breaths each for flexibility and stability.

- Cool down with wrist circles.

**Day 17:**

- Warm up with head circles.

- Move through chair tree pose, chair warrior III, and chair leg raises—holding each 8 breaths to further improve balance.

- Cool down with deep breathing.

**Day 18:**

Rest Day

## *Week 4: Strength-Building*

**Day 19:**

- Warm up with shoulder rolls.

- Do Chair sit-ups (5), Deep chair squats (5), and close with chair sun salutations. Repeat this three times.

- Cool down with wrist and ankle rolls.

**Day 20:**

- Warm up with neck rolls.

- Practice chair push-ups, seated jumping jacks, and seated leg raises—15 reps each for strengthening the full body.

- Cool down with wrist stretches.

**Day 21:**

- Warm up with arm circles.

- Hold isometric abdominal squeezes, chair dips, and seated side raises—15 seconds each to develop endurance.

- Cool down with ankle and wrist rolls.

**Day 22:**

- Warm up with gentle backbends.

- Start with single leg forward bend (do both sides), your triangle pose, and end with a half-sun salutation. Repeat this flow three times.

- Cool down with deep breathing.

**Day 23:**

- Warm up with shoulder shrugs.

- Move through chair push-ups, and chair squats—20 reps each to build strength and aerobic capacity.

- Cool down with meditation.

**Day 24:**

- Warm up with ankle rolls.

- Move through seated mountain pose, seated forward fold, and seated tree pose— hold each of these for 8 to 10 breaths. Repeat the flow three times with short breaks in between before cooling down.

- Cool down with figure 4 stretch.

**Day 25:**

- Warm up with seated cat- cow pose.

- Perform resistance band exercises, rows, bicep curls, squats with overhead presses—12 reps each to challenge muscular strength.

- Cool down with ankle rotations.

**Day 26: Review Day**

- Warm up, then practice your 4-5 favorite poses and exercises from previous weeks, holding each 5-8 breaths.

- Cool down with deep breathing.

**Day 27: Review Day**

- Warm up, then move through another 4-5 favorite poses and exercises, holding each for 5-8 breaths.

- Cool down with meditation.

**Bonus Day 28: Heart Health**

- Warm up with shoulder shrugs and arm circles.

- Practice seated backbend, chair twist, seated side bend, and palm tree pose—holding each 8-10 breaths to open the chest and improve heart health.

- Cool down with alternate nostril breathing.

# Conclusion

The word yoga itself means "to yoke" or "to unite." So I hope that you were able to unite or piece back together the parts that felt out of place, or that you're at the very least on your way there.

As you complete this journey, reflect on the aspects of yourself that you've been able to bring into greater harmony—your mind, body, and spirit. The gentle poses and breathing exercises were designed not just to increase strength and flexibility, but to foster a deeper sense of integration. If you struggled at times, that's perfectly normal. The path of yoga is one of patience, compassion, and non-judgment toward yourself. Even the most experienced practitioners have days when their minds wander or their bodies don't quite cooperate. What matters most is that you showed up, you did your best in that moment, and you'll have another opportunity tomorrow.

The uniting principles of yoga extend far beyond the physical practice. Maybe you've noticed a newfound ability to be more present throughout your day, less reactive to stressors, and kinder toward yourself and others. Or maybe you've rediscovered an inner resilience that helps you flow through life's inevitable changes with more grace.

These are all signs that the tools of chair yoga are taking root within you, slowly calming the turbulent waters of the mind and allowing your most authentic, peaceful self to resurface. As you continue this journey, have faith that the unifying effects will continue to blossom in beautifully unexpected ways.

At its essence, yoga reminds us that we are all already whole, already complete - the disparate pieces were never actually separate. Your role is simply to peel away the layers of conditioning that have accumulated over the years and obscured that truth. Chair yoga clears the window so you can more clearly see and accept your perfectly imperfect, unified self. Embrace the growth you've experienced, while also understanding that this evolution is an eternal process of becoming more coherently and joyfully you. Let this be a 🔲🔲🔲🔲🔲🔲🔲🔲 🔲🔲🔲🔲🔲, not an ending point. Continue exploring yoga's unifying pathways of movement, breath, meditation, and wisdom. Where they will ultimately lead you is to the profound recognition that you've contained the answers all along. That is the supreme yoga - and my biggest wish for you.

# Exercises List

Made in the USA
Middletown, DE
08 January 2025

69086053R00064